VEGGIE
LEAN IN 15

JOE WICKS
THE BODY COACH

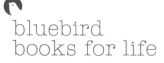

First published 2018 by Bluebird
an imprint of Pan Macmillan
20 New Wharf Road, London N1 9RR
Associated companies throughout the world
www.panmacmillan.com

ISBN 978-1-5098-5615-2

Food photography © Maja Smend
All other photography © Glen Burrows
Illustrations: Shutterstock

Credits
Publisher: Carole Tonkinson
Senior Editor: Martha Burley
Design: Ami Smithson
Food Styling: Bianca Nice
Prop Styling: Lydia Brun

9 8 7 6 5 4 3 2 1

A CIP catalogue record for this book is available from the British Library.
Printed and bound in Italy.

Designed and Typeset by www.cabinlondon.co.uk

Visit **www.panmacmillan.com** to read more about all our books and to
buy them. You will also find features, author interviews and news of any
author events, and you can sign up for e-newsletters so that you're
always first to hear about our new releases.

bluebird
books for life

Contents

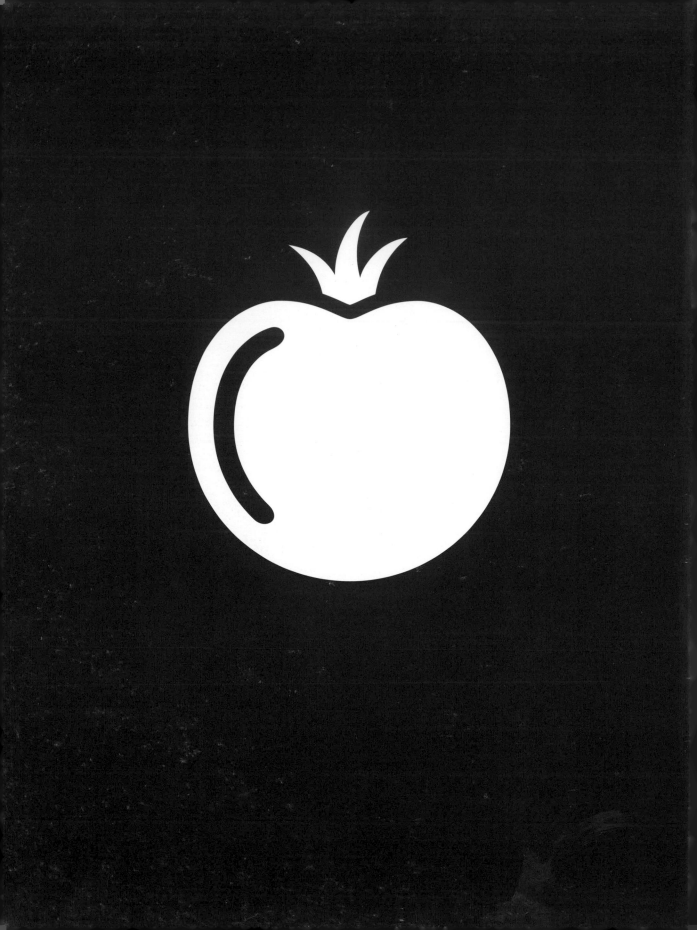

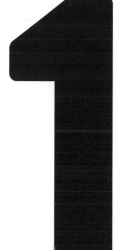

INTRODUCTION

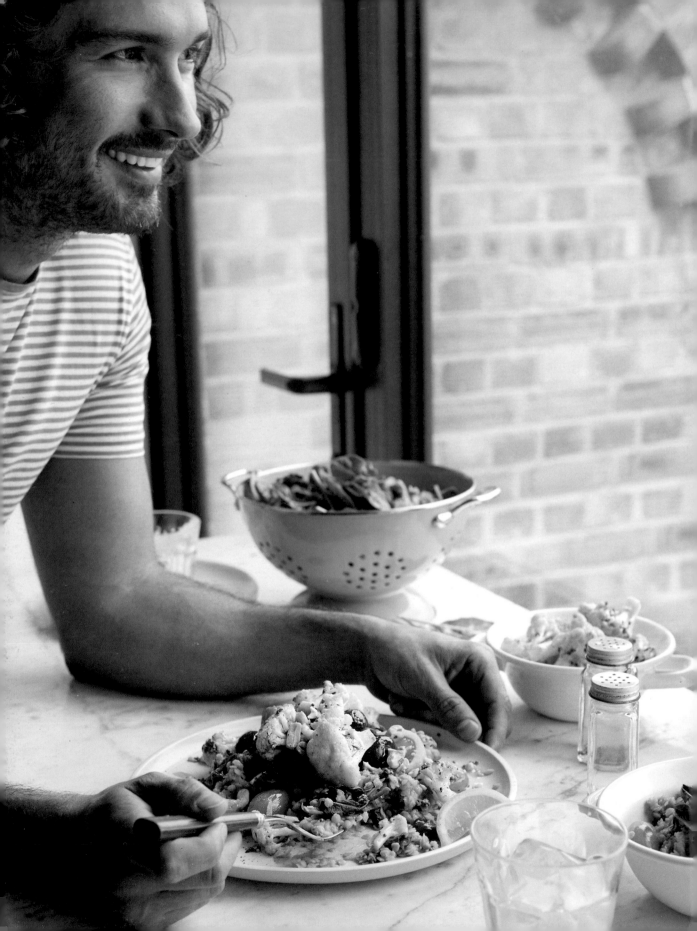

If you had asked me five years ago, back when I was a personal trainer, if I would ever write a vegetarian book, I would have said 'No chance – veggie food is boring', or 'Nah, I don't believe being a veggie is healthy, because you can't get enough protein', but here I am: a bit more grown-up, and way more educated on the subject.

From the outset, I want to be completely honest and open with you. I am not a vegetarian or vegan. I still enjoy a steak and a burger now and again, and truthfully I'm not sure if I will ever give those up completely. There are trendy new phrases like 'flexitarian' or 'reducitarian' flying about, but I don't think labels are all that helpful, or that we should put ourselves under any pressure to fit into a particular group. Some days I eat meat, other days I don't. All I know is I'm enjoying veggie food more than ever, and I'm excited to share these new recipes and workouts with you.

It has been a gradual change. I haven't watched any of the pro-vegan documentaries or read any books on the environment that have 'shocked' me into not eating meat. I suppose I've just become more aware of the impact my own food choices have on my health and the environment.

Like many people, I've sensed a natural shift in my attitude towards vegetarian and plant-based food, and this education has been shaped online by YouTube, Facebook and Instagram, where people are very vocal about lifestyle choices and views on animal welfare, global warming and the environment.

Another big factor that's prompted me to eat more veggie food is the incredible dishes I've tasted in the past couple of years, as so many restaurants now cater for vegetarians and vegans. I used to think veggie recipes were all boring salads and quinoa, but the more I experiment, the more I see how totally wrong that view is. Veggie food can be easy, delicious and satisfying when done well, and that's what this book is all about. The recipes have the speed and simplicity you'll be familiar with from my old-school Lean in 15 books, with all the same great taste and flavour.

> ❛I'm enjoying veggie food more than ever, and I'm excited to share these new recipes with you❜

> **'Veggie food can be easy, delicious and satisfying when done well, and that's what this book is all about '**

And I've discovered that with a little thought and preparation, you can definitely stay lean and get enough protein with a veggie diet.

Like so many other people, I'm beginning to be more aware of the issues around sustainability. A few years ago, I would never have questioned whether my fish was sustainably sourced or considered that the palm oil used in my favourite peanut butter was destroying thousands of miles of forests in Indonesia and along with it all the wildlife that inhabits it. And I see how eating lower down on the food chain (plants rather than meat) can add up to fewer carbon emissions.

But it's not only what we eat: it's also how we shop. We can get loose fruit and veg in a paper bag or go for avocados packed in double plastic. With the campaigns to ban plastic straws and single-use water bottles, I've started to really think about the effect of plastic in our oceans. We are used to buying food all neatly presented in trays with plastic wrappers, and when we chuck those in the recycling container, we don't really think about what it means in the long term. The plastic doesn't get recycled the way most of us think it does. The dustman comes and takes it all to landfill sites where it takes hundreds of years to degrade. There is no way that this is going to work in the long term.

It's been my own decision and my own journey to reach this point. And one thing I know is that my attitude and mindset towards nutrition and my purchasing choices has changed and continues to change as I grow and learn more.

I think that's a really important thing to remember: don't be pressured by anyone to conform to a certain diet or lifestyle. It's your choice to make and how you feel about it today may be very different to this time next year. I believe that we are on a journey, and, in the future, all of us will move towards eating more vegetarian food, out of choice and also out of necessity. I hope this book can help inspire you to give veggie food a go and that it will have a positive impact on your health and our environment.

A close friend of mine who is a vegan and really passionate about protecting our world once said to me, 'Joe, you have a huge audience and a platform to really make a change, you should use that power to influence people in a positive way.' At the time I didn't really think I could make a difference – or maybe if I'm honest I didn't care enough

– but that's changed now. I realize that millions of people cook my food and I can be a positive influence, and be part of the solution. That same friend also said to me, 'Joe, it's the ritual of eating meat that you love, not the actual meat itself.' At the time, I didn't really understand what she meant, but the more veggie food I cook, the more I understand what she means. Now that I'm creating really quick, tasty and satisfying veggie meals, I realize that I don't miss the meat. I love a burger, but a peri-peri halloumi burger makes a nice change (see page 54). It's still a burger.

Lately, more and more of my followers have been engaging with my vegetarian recipes and I always really listen to my followers to understand what people like and are looking for. When I tried to share a few veggie recipes a couple of years ago, there just wasn't a demand. However, in the last year, as I've started to love eating more veggie stuff, people have been going crazy for the veggie recipes I've shared. I've also seen a shift in my audience, and this certainly helped me to be more confident that now is the time to release a veggie book.

Veggie Lean in 15 is the 'veggie book for the meat lover'. I've worked hard to create recipes that taste good and are so satisfying that you don't even question where the meat is. I've taken all the foods I love and 'veggified' them.

So, thank you for buying *Veggie Lean in 15*. Good luck with it! Get stuck in and see how much you love the recipes. Not only are you going to get fitter and healthier, you'll also know you are doing your little bit to keep our planet healthy now and for the future.

Lots of Love, Joe

UNDERSTANDING THE BASICS

I'm going to talk a little about the basics of nutrition to help you understand the importance of fuelling your body correctly. My philosophy on health, fitness and nutrition has always been consistent. I like to keep things simple and achievable, so you can follow it, enjoy it and sustain it.

For those who follow me online or own one of my previous books, you'll know that unlike some diets, I don't promote calorie-counting or macro-tracking. I think it's an unnecessary pressure, which can result in an unhealthy relationship with food and exercise. It is also unrealistic to think that people can track, count and hit a certain target every day – especially as every day is different. Some days you'll be more active than others, some days you will forget your prepped lunch and eat out, so I believe in a much more flexible and enjoyable way of making progress.

I want to encourage you to focus on the basics and keep stuff really simple. This means easy home-cooking, regular home-workouts and small, positive lifestyle changes. By doing these things consistently and cutting out processed junk foods, you will naturally create an energy deficit and therefore start to burn fat.

Creating an energy or calorie deficit means you are burning more energy than you are consuming, and we know this is essential for fat loss. The important thing to remember is that you do not need to 'count calories' in order to be in a calorie deficit. Just by living a healthier lifestyle, becoming more active and making better food choices, energy deficit becomes a by-product. It's a 'win win' as you will look better, live better and most of all feel better.

Another reason I don't include the calorie content in my recipes is because you are totally unique and your body has its own unique energy demands. This is influenced by your metabolism, lean body mass, age, physical activity levels, hormones and other factors. This means there is no perfect daily calorie intake or ideal portion size for fat loss. I want you to use the recipes in this book as a guide, but based on how you feel or how active you are, adjust the portions accordingly. Put simply, this means if you are a fit and active 25-year-old, training hard five days per week and doing manual labour, you will need more food than a less active 50-year-old office-worker doing yoga three days per week.

If you really want to give this plan a go, my advice is to follow the workouts and make the recipes as they are listed in the book. Then if you feel like the portions are too big or too small you can adjust them the next time round. You don't need to over-think this part or get stressed out by it. Just eat to feel energized. If you feel full up and satisfied, then you are probably doing just great.

Keep in mind that I'm not a fan of low-calorie diets so the portions are generous. This is because I want you to exercise. I want you to be active rather than sedentary. I want you to burn fat and build lean muscle through resistance and HIIT training. This means your body needs to be fuelled, and eating like a rabbit isn't going to achieve that. So enjoy the energy these meals give you and work hard in your sessions.

How do we get energy?

Our body gets energy from three sources, known as macronutrients: fat, protein and carbohydrates. They all play an important role in our bodies and a good balance of all of them is essential for optimal health. You do not need to completely cut out any of these in order to burn fat. There are a lot of misconceptions in nutrition for fat loss. One common misconception is that carbohydrates make you gain fat – in fact, carbohydrates are an important fuel-source for muscle repair and growth. We gain and store excess body fat when we are eating in a calorie surplus and this plan is going to help you avoid that so you can get lean and stay lean.

Over the next few pages, I've put together a guide to each macronutrient, including information about their function in the body and highlighting some of the best vegetarian sources.

> ❝ My portions are generous because I want you to exercise and be active, and to enjoy the energy that food gives you ❞

Protein

Essential for the growth and repair of every cell in our body including lean muscle tissue, protein also helps with regulation of metabolism, production of hormones and strengthening of our immune systems. It's very important for our health and this often leads many vegetarians to question: 'Am I getting enough protein?'. The fact is, you can be a healthy vegetarian or an unhealthy vegetarian, depending on how you eat and what nutrients you get into your diet.

When I finished my degree in Sports Science and started as a personal trainer, I used to think being a vegetarian wasn't healthy due to the lack of complete protein sources available. (A complete protein source is one that contains all of the essential amino acids needed by the body, such as animal protein sources.)

The main rationale for this was my belief that as a veggie you simply could not get enough protein in your diet, especially if you trained hard and frequently like myself. This was reinforced by my nutrition studies during my personal trainer course and magazines and journals that constantly reinforce the importance of getting enough protein in your diet. Chicken, steak and fish served with brown rice: it was on repeat.

All of my knowledge at that time was based on the culture of building muscle. I just didn't believe that you could build a strong muscular physique out of spinach, quinoa and sweet potato. So I carried on as I was, eating animal protein sources three times a day, every day. Eggs for breakfast, chicken for lunch and steak or fish for dinner.

In reality, for years there have been vegetarian and vegan fitness models and trainers with incredible physiques all over the world. I just hadn't been looking in that direction and stayed in the meat-eating camp.

The fact is, you won't consume as much protein every day using this veggie book as opposed to using my first Lean in 15 books, but that doesn't mean you will not get through enough protein or be as healthy.

❛These recipes include a wide variety of protein sources to ensure you get enough protein and stay healthy❜

I've worked hard to create recipes that include a wide variety of protein sources to ensure you will be getting enough protein. There are some awesome vegetarian sources such as soya, buckwheat and quinoa that are 'complete' and contain all the essential amino acids. Protein is also found in smaller quantities in vegetables, grains and pulses and in order to get all of your essential amino acids you just have to be a bit smart by combining different sources. Below is a list of protein-rich vegetarian sources that you can find throughout the book.

Protein-rich sources

- **Beans and pulses** Lentils, chickpeas, black beans, kidney beans
- **Grains** Oats, barley, rice, quinoa
- **Dairy** Milk, cheese, Greek yoghurt
- **Eggs**
- **Soya and tofu**
- **Nuts and seeds** Almonds, cashews, chia seeds, flaxseeds, nut butters
- **Vegetables** Green peas, broccoli, spinach, asparagus, artichokes, potatoes, sweet potatoes, Brussels sprouts

As you can see, there are plenty of protein sources and this means your meals can be varied and tasty, and you don't need to rely on Quorn or tofu every day of the week.

One important aspect of protein intake when you're losing weight is that it has the ability to reduce appetite. Protein keeps you feeling full much better than fat and carbohydrates so this means creating that energy deficit can be easier and more sustainable.

Carbohydrates

Being a vegetarian often means you will consume a higher amount of carbohydrates in the form of rice, oats, lentils, quinoa, pasta and fruit. Do not fear this, or think you can't get lean, because you can. Remember carbs are the body's preferred source of energy during high-intensity exercise and as long as you're burning more energy than you consume, you will burn body fat. Carbohydrates also help repair and rebuild muscle tissue damaged during exercise.

Many people don't get enough fibrous carbohydrates in their diet, but with this plan you certainly will. Unlike starchy and sugary carbohydrates, fibrous carbohydrates are not digested by the body. Non-fibrous carbohydrates elevate your blood sugar levels and provide calories, while fibre does not. This means you can eat loads of veg without having to keep track or worry about over-consumption. Vegetables are the best sources of fibrous carbohydrates. Eating more fibre will improve your intestinal health and digestion so being a veggie is good for you. Here is a list of good sources of carbohydrates that you can find throughout the recipes in the book.

Good sources of carbs

- **Vegetables** Carrots, butternut squash, spinach, peppers, mushrooms, sweet potatoes, potatoes
- **Fruits** Berries, bananas, apples, oranges, pears, grapes, mango, pineapples
- **Legumes** Black beans, kidney beans, chickpeas, butterbeans, white beans, soya beans, quinoa
- **Whole grains** Wholemeal bread, wholewheat pasta, oats, barley, brown rice, buckwheat

As you can see, several of the carbohydrate sources listed above also feature in the protein section. This means your body is getting good sources of both from a variety of different foods which is a big bonus for your weekly eating plan.

Fat

The most energy-dense macronutrient of all, just one gram of fat provides over double the energy of a gram of protein or carbohydrate. This makes fat a brilliant source of energy, but one that needs to be considered more carefully when it comes to a balanced diet and creating an energy deficit. For example, just because homemade almond butter is healthy doesn't mean you can eat a tub of the stuff every day. It is just about enjoying the different sources in sensible quantities throughout your meals.

Fats often taste so damn good – whether in the form of nut butters, cheese, olive oil, butter or avocados – but it is there for more than just taste.

Fats provide energy, help the body absorb fat-soluble vitamins, help produce essential hormones in the body and also help with the maintenance of healthy hair, skin and nails. This means fat is not optional, but essential for good health, and that's why I don't agree with very low-fat diets.

However, there are different types of fat, so here is a list of some healthy fat sources in my recipes.

Good sources of fat

- **Olives**
- **Cheese**
- **Butter**
- **Eggs**
- **Coconut oil**
- **Olive oil**
- **Nuts**
- **Avocados**
- **Yoghurt**
- **Seeds**

How to create a calorie deficit

I don't know how many calories I eat every day and I'm not going to start counting now. I want you to start eating intuitively and learn to create your energy deficit through portion sizes and home-cooking combined with exercise.

If you think back to years ago, when our grandparents hadn't even heard of the word 'calorie' and nutritional science didn't exist, we all did just fine. We didn't have a diabetes and obesity epidemic. We just cooked a lot more at home. This was before the invention of fast food and convenience-processed food products.

The fact is, we are all up against it now. At every turn there are unhealthy on-the-go foods that are high in sugar and the wrong sorts of fats. There's a petrol station, corner shop or supermarket ready to sell us crap. Not only that, but there's also a constant reminder with adverts on the bus stops, train stations and Instagram feeds that there is processed food ready to grab and go.

Products made to make our life 'easier' are slowly but surely making us more and more unhealthy, sick and overweight. Do your best to aim to remove these types of unhealthy foods from your diet. Now of course I'm not talking about a

'Make small changes and introduce good habits '

lifetime ban on chocolate – oh god no, that would be awful!
But just allow them as a weekly treat rather than a daily reward.

My next challenge for you is to start to incorporate the workouts into your week. Just four to five workouts per week really will change your life. It's going to allow you to enjoy your food while feeling energized, happy and confident.

On days that you are more active and smash a workout you can just eat a bit more and on days you rest or are sedentary just eat mindfully and fuel your body accordingly. Treat your body like a sexy Italian sports car. Put the best fuel in it you possibly can without over filling the tank or letting it run out of fuel. Both will damage the engine and your chassis in the end.

So there it is. Not as complicated or as scary as it seems, is it? Make small changes, introduce good habits, prep your own food more and exercise regularly. That's how I create my energy deficit and how I stay lean, and I'm confident you can do the same.

How should I be eating on this plan?

If you want to follow this book as an actual full veggie plan, then go for it. If, like me, you still want to eat some meat or fish during the week, then you can simply use the recipes in this book to give you ideas of quick and tasty veggie meals to incorporate into your diet – however it best suits you and your lifestyle.

You may want to join the popular Meat-Free Monday movement, whereby you eat veggie on Mondays. Or you could aim to eat one or two veggie meals a day and one with an animal protein source.

I personally love to eat out in restaurants for a chargrilled steak or rack of ribs, as I don't cook those for myself at home. While at home I'm starting to make swaps and eat veggie.

My meal plan is very simple to follow and flexible: aim to eat three meals from any section of the book each day, and up to two snacks if you need them. There are no set meal eating times so simply eat at any point of the day which suits you and fits into your lifestyle. You can also exercise any time of the day. You can eat before a workout or, if you prefer, train fasted (on an empty stomach) and eat afterwards. As long as you train hard, eat decent portion sizes and mix up your meal choices you will get a good variety of protein sources and nutrients to maintain a strong and lean body.

Ultimately there is no perfect diet for everyone. You need to find what works well for you and your lifestyle and body. You may be someone who feels full of energy and super healthy eating only vegetarian food, or you could be someone who feels a bit lethargic and needs to eat one red meat or fish meal a day or a week.

You just need to eat in a way which makes you happy, feel energized, sleep well and have good digestion. I don't think you need to feel any pressure to be too extreme either way. It's about finding that healthy, happy middle-ground. Even by eating one extra veggie meal a day you are getting healthier and impacting the environment in a positive way.

Hydration

Another really important thing to consider when trying to get lean is good hydration. Most people don't drink enough and often being thirsty can lead to people thinking they are hungry and unnecessarily snacking. Aim to drink 2–4 litres of water per day. This will help with your digestion, energy levels and also ensure your body is more efficient at metabolizing fat.

Sleep and wellbeing

One of the most under-utilized tools for good health and wellbeing is sleep. I know it can be difficult with work and family commitments, but try to prioritize sleep as it really is transformative. A good night's sleep will allow you to wake up rested and energized enough to really put some effort into your workouts. It will also give you better focus and productivity so you can achieve more.

Try to get into a regular routine where you get a decent night's sleep every night. Around 7–8 hours would be ideal. It may mean turning Netflix off an hour early, but it will be worth it in the morning!

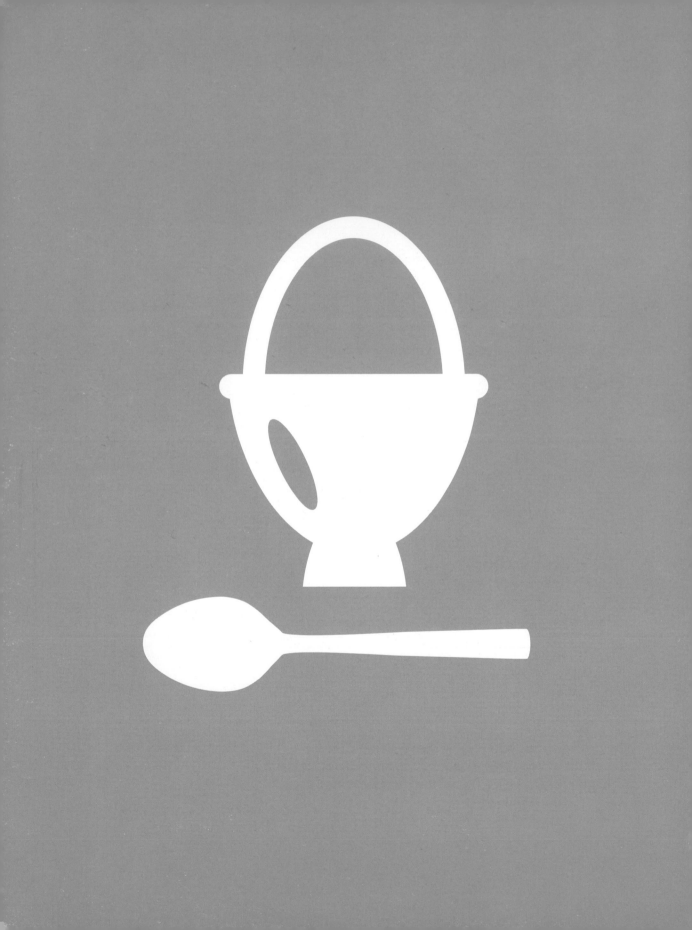

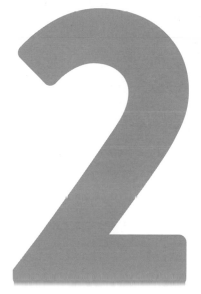

2

ALL-DAY
BREAKFASTS

SERVES 1

Protein power pancakes

Ingredients

1 large banana
¼ tsp ground cinnamon
seeds of 1 cardamom pod
1 egg
2 tbsp almond butter
3 tbsp rolled oats
¼ tsp bicarbonate of soda
½ tbsp coconut oil
drizzle of maple syrup, to serve

Method

Roughly chop half the banana and place in the blender with the rest of the pancake ingredients apart from the coconut oil and maple syrup. Blitz to a smooth batter.

Melt the coconut oil in a decent non-stick frying pan over a medium heat. Spoon the batter into the pan to make three pancakes, leaving some room between each one as they will spread a little. Fry the pancakes for about 1 minute on each side. You will know when it is time to flip because little bubbles will appear all over the surface of the pancake.

Slice up the remaining banana. Stack the pancakes on top of each other with a few pieces of banana between each pancake. Drizzle with a little maple syrup and serve.

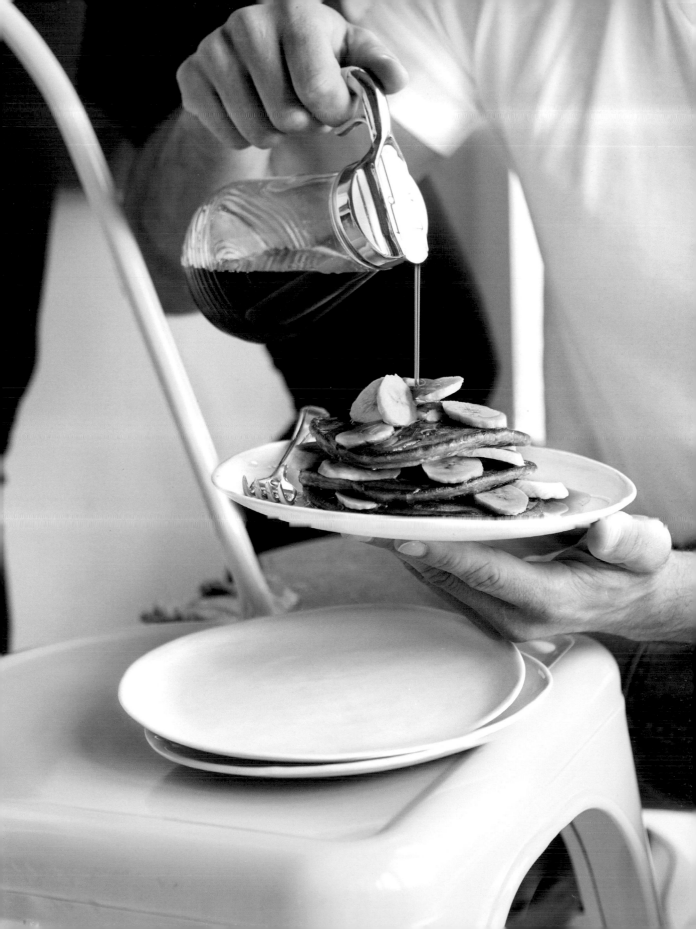

MAKES 500G

VE

Joe's spiced nutty granola

LONGER RECIPE
MAKE AHEAD
Keep in an airtight
container for up to 2 weeks.

Ingredients

2 tbsp coconut oil
3 tbsp maple syrup
250g mixed nuts – I like
  cashews, pecans, walnuts
  and almonds
100g pumpkin seeds
150g rolled oats
1 tsp ground cinnamon
1 tsp ground ginger
salt

Method

Preheat the oven to 160°C (fan 140°C, gas mark 3).
Melt the coconut oil in a large bowl in the microwave.

Mix in the rest of the ingredients along with a good
pinch of salt, then tip the granola out onto a large, flat
baking sheet. Spread out into a single layer.

Bake for 35 minutes, mixing everything around every
now and then so that the granola toasts evenly.

Remove from the oven and leave to cool. Serve a portion
in a bowl with your choice of milk or yoghurt.

JOE'S TOP TIP Baking the granola for a little bit more
time at a lower temperature toasts the nuts
evenly, bringing out their sweetness.

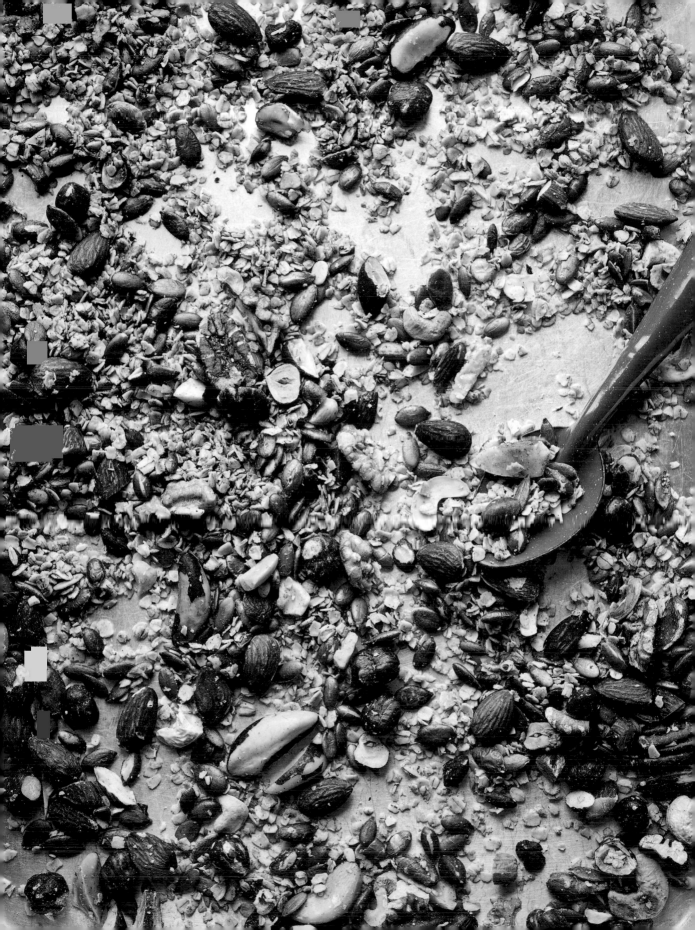

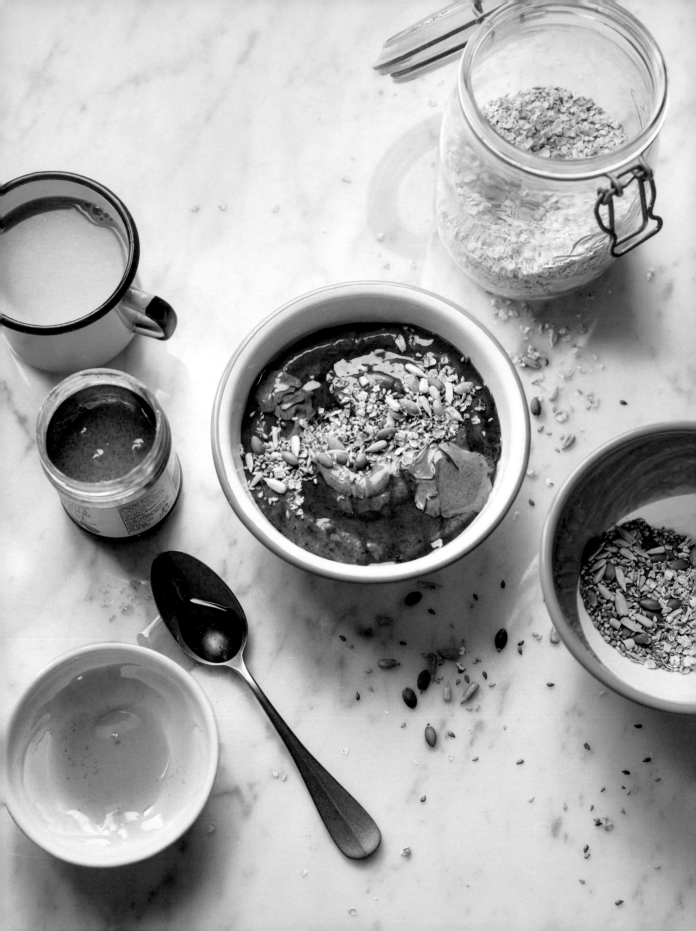

SERVES 1

MAKE AHEAD
You can blitz the fruit and yoghurt the night before and keep it in the fridge.

Ingredients

½ avocado, flesh scooped out
1 small banana, roughly chopped
2 handfuls of mixed frozen berries
2 tbsp natural yoghurt
1½ tbsp rolled oats
1½ tbsp mixed seeds
1 tbsp almond butter
drizzle of honey

Avo and berry breakfast pot

Method

Place the avocado, banana, frozen berries and natural yoghurt in a blender and blitz with a splash of water until smooth. Tip into a bowl or pot to take to work.

In a dry frying pan over a medium heat, toast the oats and seeds until the seeds start to pop. Take off the heat.

When you're ready to eat, top the avocado berry pot with the toasted oats and seeds, almond butter and a drizzle of honey.

MAKE AHEAD
You can keep the batter for
up to 1 hour in the fridge.

Ingredients

2 tbsp desiccated coconut

¼ tsp bicarbonate of soda

1 scoop (30g) chocolate
   protein powder

3 tbsp coconut milk

1 egg

1 tsp cocoa powder (over
   70% cocoa solids)

salt

30g dark chocolate, chopped
   or grated into shards

½ tbsp coconut oil

dollop of coconut yoghurt,
   to serve

Bangin' bounty pancakes

Method

To make the batter, whizz up the desiccated coconut, bicarbonate of soda, protein powder, coconut milk, egg and cocoa powder in a blender along with a pinch of salt. Stir through three-quarters of the chopped chocolate.

Melt the coconut oil in a large non-stick frying pan over a medium heat. Spoon in the batter to make three pancakes. Fry the pancakes for about 1 minute on each side. You will know when it is time to flip because little bubbles will appear all over the surface.

Pile the pancakes on top of each other, top with a dollop of coconut yoghurt and the remaining chocolate. Winning.

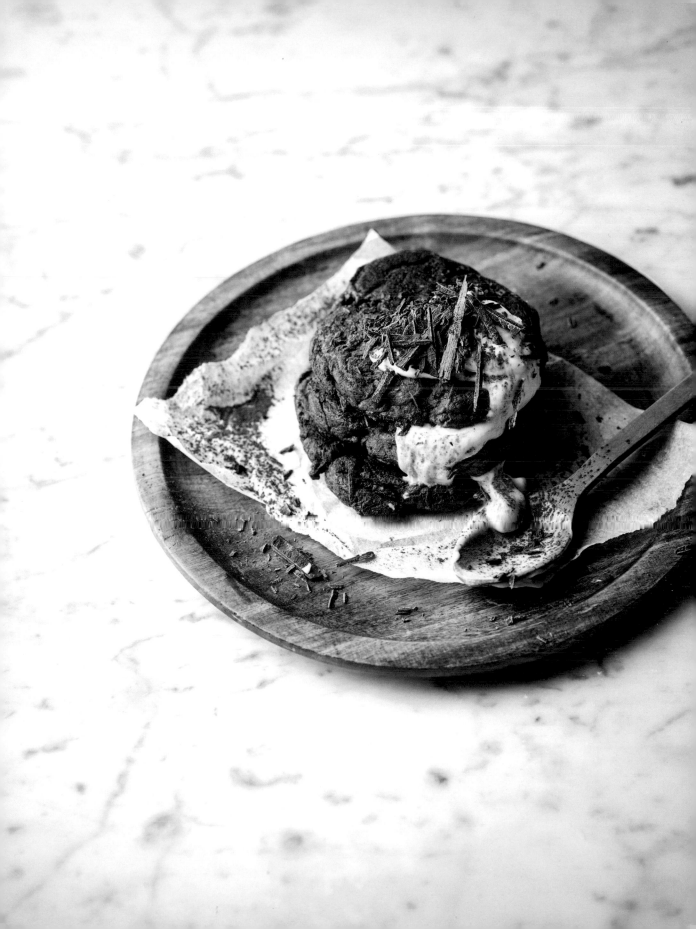

SERVES 1

LONGER RECIPE
MAKE AHEAD

Ingredients

75g rolled oats
1 carrot, peeled and grated
¼ tsp mixed spice
1 scoop (30g) vanilla protein powder
200ml almond milk
20g pecans
2 tbsp Greek yoghurt
drizzle of honey

Carrot cake overnight oats

Method

Tip all the ingredients apart from the pecans, yoghurt and honey into a bowl and stir well. Pour the mixture into a sealable container and leave to soak in the fridge overnight.

When you're ready to eat, toast the pecans in a dry frying pan over a medium heat until smelling nutty, then allow to cool and roughly chop.

Remove the lid from your overnight oats, top with the yoghurt, sprinkle over the toasted pecans and drizzle with honey.

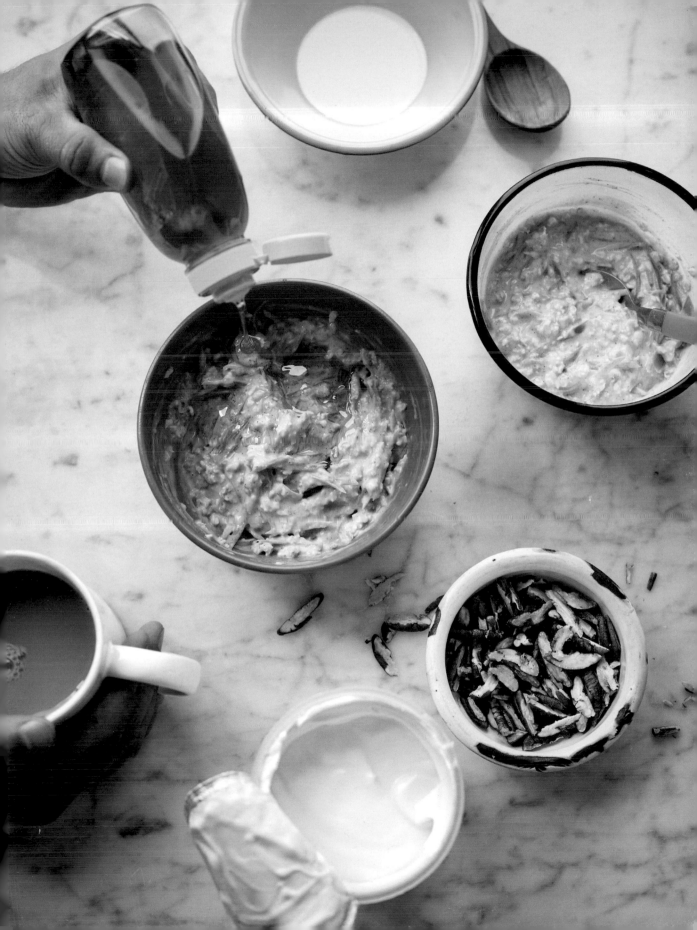

**SERVES
2**

Ingredients

1 tbsp butter, plus extra
   for greasing
120g rolled oats, plus 2 tbsp
2 scoops (60g) vanilla protein
   powder
100g mixed berries – I like
   strawberries and blueberries
400ml almond milk
salt
1 tbsp honey
2 tbsp pumpkin seeds
2 tbsp flaked almonds

Baked berry crumble porridge

Method

Preheat the oven to 190°C (fan 170°C, gas mark 5). Use
a little bit of butter to lightly grease a large baking dish.

Pour 120g rolled oats into the baking dish with the protein
powder and stir well to combine. Add the berries, almond
milk and a pinch of salt. Put the porridge in the oven to bake
for 15 minutes, until most of the liquid has been absorbed
and the top of the porridge has set.

Meanwhile, ping the butter with the honey in the microwave
in a small bowl for a few seconds until the butter has melted
then mix in the remaining 2 tablespoons of oats, the pumpkin
seeds and flaked almonds.

After 15 minutes of cooking, sprinkle the crumble mixture
over the porridge and return to the oven for a further
5 minutes until the porridge is thick and creamy.
(Pictured overleaf.)

SERVES 1

Cinnamon porridge with quick berry compote

Ingredients

2 handfuls of frozen berries
1 tsp maple syrup
75g rolled oats
¼ tsp ground cinnamon
250ml almond milk
salt
1 scoop (30g) vanilla protein powder

Method

First make the quick berry compote. Tip the frozen berries and the maple syrup into a small saucepan over a medium heat. Cook for 3 minutes until the berries have collapsed and look jammy. Turn off the heat.

Put the oats, cinnamon, 100ml water and three-quarters of the almond milk into a saucepan along with a pinch of salt. Bring to the boil, then turn down the heat. Cook the porridge for 4–5 minutes, stirring regularly until creamy.

Mix the remaining almond milk with the protein powder to get rid of any lumps, then add to the pan. Give everything a good stir, then put back on the heat for 30 seconds to warm through.

Spoon the porridge into your bowl and top with the quick berry compote. (Pictured overleaf.)

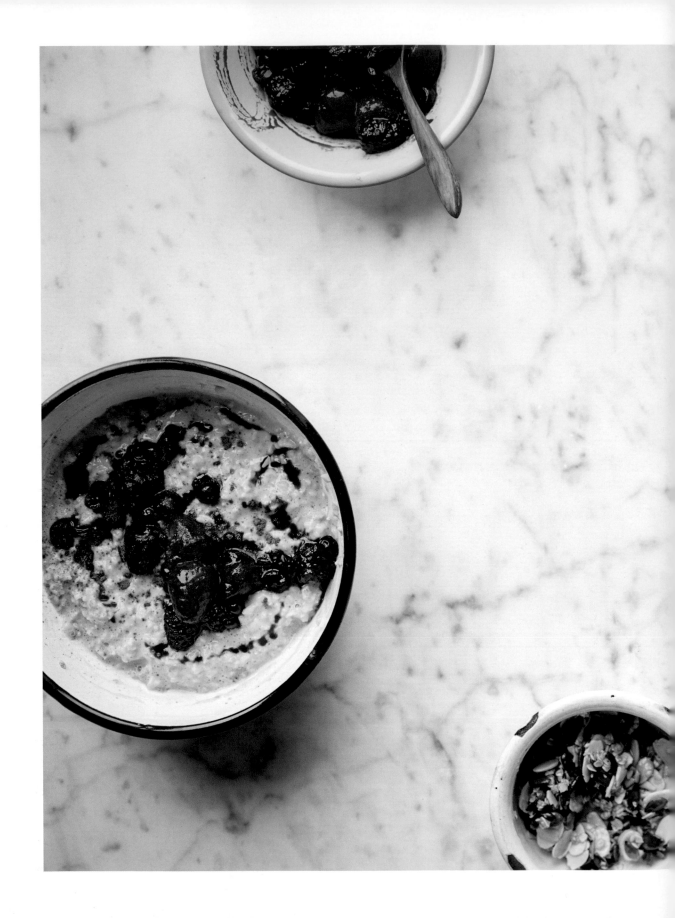

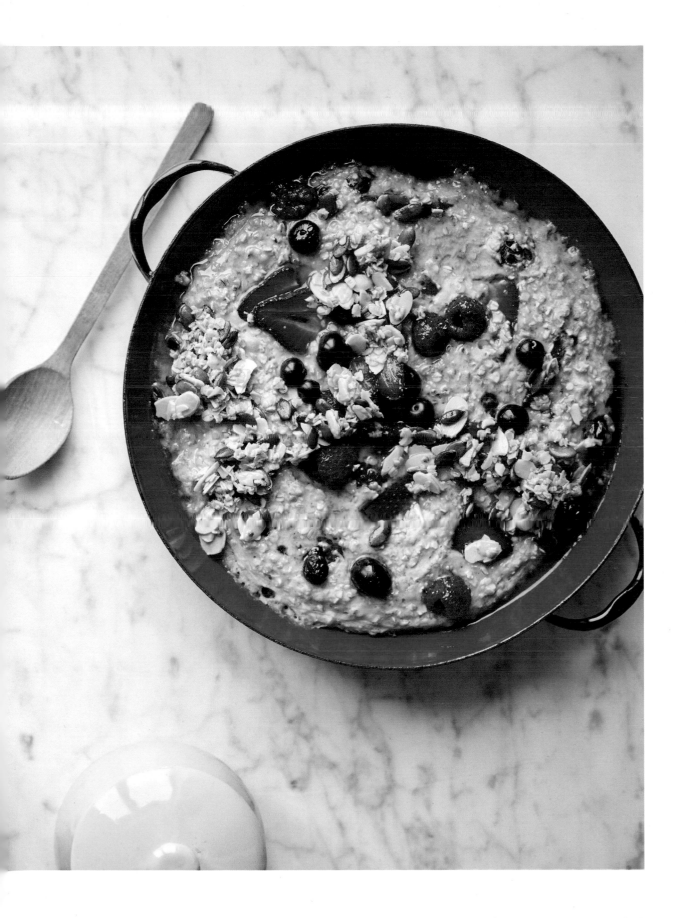

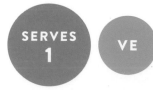

SERVES 1 · **VE**

Mango, pineapple and cashew smoothie

Ingredients

2 tbsp cashew butter
75g mango chunks
75g frozen pineapple chunks
big pinch of ground turmeric
black pepper

Method

Place all the ingredients in a blender with 150ml water and a crack of black pepper. Blitz until smooth. (Pictured overleaf.)

SERVES 1

Kiwi, apple and ginger smoothie

Ingredients

1 kiwi, peeled and roughly
  chopped
½ avocado, flesh scooped out
small piece of ginger, peeled and
  roughly chopped
1 small apple, cored and
  roughly chopped
large handful of baby
  spinach leaves
1 scoop (30g) vanilla protein
  powder

Method

Place all the ingredients in a blender with 150ml water and blitz until smooth. (Pictured overleaf.)

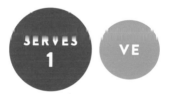

SERVES 1 **VE**

Peanut butter, oat and banana smoothie

Ingredients

1 ripe banana, roughly
  chopped
2 tbsp peanut butter
250ml almond milk
50g porridge oats

Method

Place all the ingredients in a blender and blitz until smooth. (Pictured overleaf.)

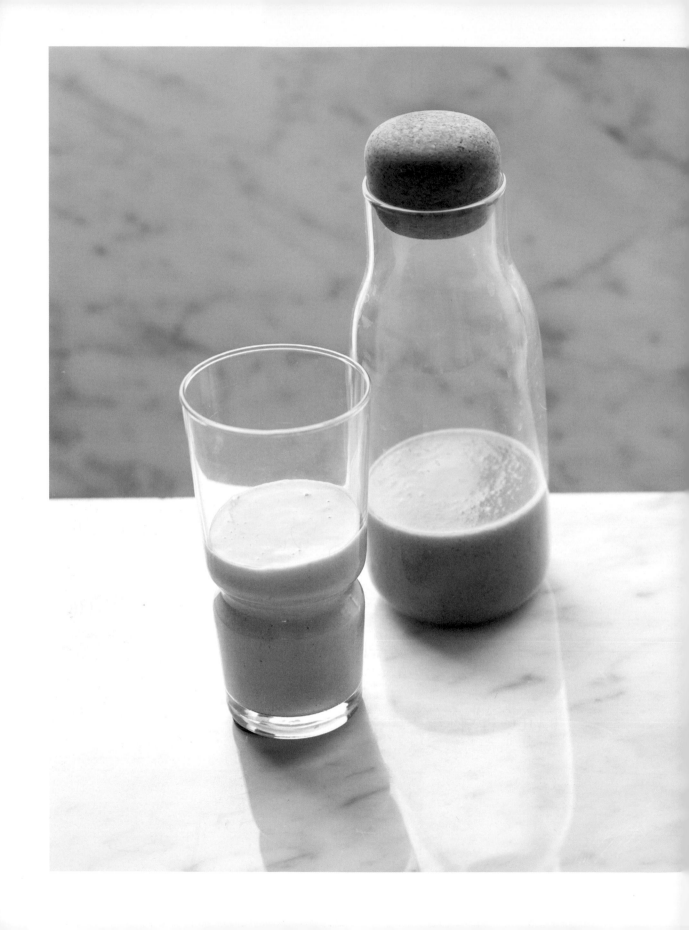

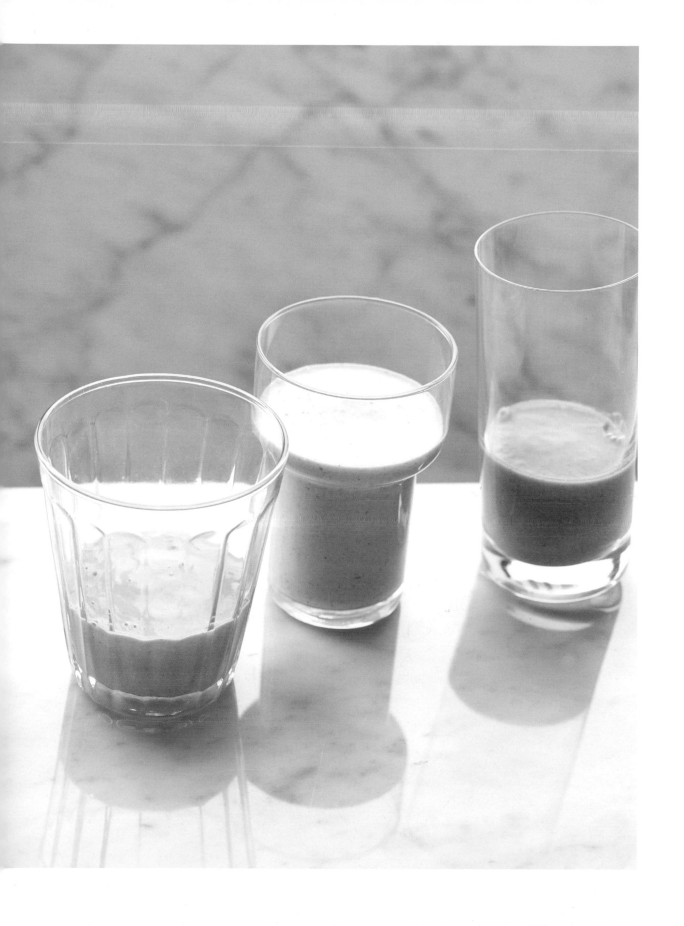

SERVES 1

Herby spinach, spring onion and cheddar frittata

MAKE AHEAD
Enjoy hot or cold.

Ingredients

3 eggs
1 tbsp dill, finely chopped
1 tbsp parsley, finely chopped
pinch of dried chilli flakes
50g cheddar, grated
salt and pepper
1 tbsp coconut oil
2 spring onions, finely sliced
2 large handfuls of baby
  spinach leaves
green salad, to serve

Method

Preheat your grill to maximum.

Crack the eggs into a bowl, whisk with a fork then add the dill, parsley, chilli flakes, three-quarters of the grated cheddar and a good pinch of salt and pepper.

Melt the coconut oil in a small ovenproof non-stick frying pan over a medium heat. Chuck in the spring onions and cook for 2 minutes until softened. Drop in the spinach and stir until wilted.

Pour in the herby egg mixture and cook for 3–4 minutes until the egg has begun to set at the sides of the pan.

Sprinkle over the remaining cheddar then slide the pan under the grill for 5 minutes until the frittata is cooked through and the top is browned.

Remove the pan from under the heat (be careful as the handle may be hot). Slide the frittata onto a plate. Serve with salad.

**SERVES
1**

Chilli, chickpea
and leek hash

Ingredients

100g new potatoes, halved
1½ tbsp coconut oil
1 leek, trimmed and sliced
salt and pepper
1 clove garlic
½ tsp fennel seeds
½ tsp chilli powder
200g chickpeas, drained
  and rinsed
2 eggs
handful of dill, roughly chopped
dollops of yoghurt, to serve

Method

Put the new potatoes in a microwaveable bowl with
1 tablespoon water. Cover with cling film then zap on
high for 5 minutes until soft.

While the potatoes are cooking, melt 1 tablespoon of the
coconut oil in a frying pan over a medium heat. Chuck in
the leek along with a pinch of salt and pepper. Cook for
5 minutes until softened.

Crush the garlic clove into the leek and stir in the fennel
seeds and chilli powder. Cook for a minute until it starts to
smell fragrant, then add the chickpeas and cooked new
potatoes. Give everything a good stir, crushing the potatoes
slightly with the back of your spoon.

Make two spaces in the chickpea–potato mix and add
in the remaining coconut oil. Allow to melt, then crack each
of the eggs into a hole and fry until the whites are set and
the yolks are runny.

Scatter over the dill, then serve the hash straight out of
the pan with a few dollops of yoghurt.

Bombay omelette

Ingredients

3 eggs
½ red onion, finely chopped
½ green chilli, finely
  chopped – remove the seeds
  if you don't like it hot
large handful of
  coriander, finely chopped
1 tomato, seeds removed and
  finely chopped
½ tsp garam masala
½ tsp coriander seeds
big pinch of ground turmeric
salt and black pepper
½ tbsp coconut oil
large handful of baby
  spinach leaves
1 tbsp toasted flaked almonds
dollop of yoghurt, to serve
  – optional

Method

Crack the eggs into a large jug. Whisk well so that the white and yolk thoroughly combine. Tip the onion, chilli, coriander, tomato, garam masala, coriander seeds and turmeric into the jug. Give everything a good stir and season with salt and pepper.

Melt the coconut oil in a small non-stick frying pan over a medium heat. Pour the egg mixture into the pan. Fry the egg, drawing in the cooked egg from the sides, for about a minute, or until it resembles scrambled egg. Spread the egg across the base of the pan to allow it to brown.

Scatter the spinach leaves over the middle of the omelette, then when you are happy that the eggs are cooked enough to hold their shape, turn off the heat and fold one half of the omelette over the spinach.

Slide the omelette onto a plate, scatter over the flaked almonds and serve with a dollop of yoghurt, if you like.

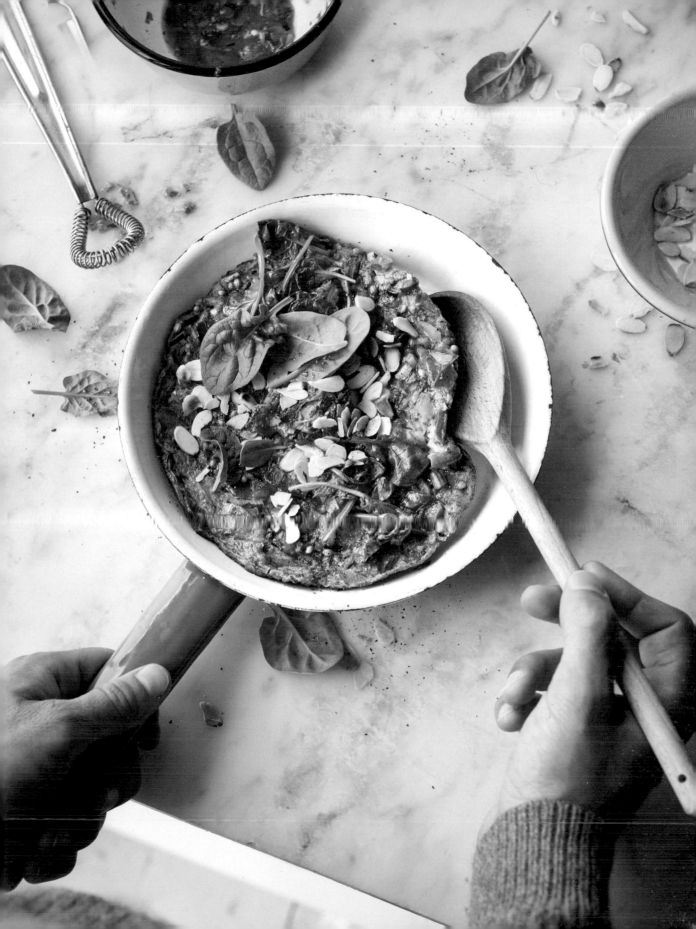

Green Turkish eggs

Ingredients

1 tbsp coconut oil, plus a smidge
2 spring onions, finely sliced
  (green bits and all)
1 clove garlic, finely chopped
100g asparagus tips, each cut
  into three pieces
2 handfuls of kale, stalks
  removed
salt and pepper
handful of mint leaves
2 eggs
½ tsp smoked paprika
2 tbsp natural yoghurt
1 tbsp toasted almonds, roughly
  chopped
crusty bread, to serve – I like
  sourdough

Method

Bring a saucepan of water to the boil.

Meanwhile, melt 1 tablespoon coconut oil in a frying pan over a medium heat. Chuck in your spring onions, garlic and asparagus. Fry for 3 minutes until the asparagus is just tender, then stir in the kale along with a good pinch of salt and pepper. When wilted, turn down the heat to its lowest to keep the greens warm. Stir through the mint leaves.

Come back to your saucepan of boiling water. Turn down the heat until the water is just 'burping'. Crack the eggs straight into the water. Poach for 3–4 minutes or until the white has set but the yolk is still runny, then carefully lift out with a slotted spoon and drain on kitchen roll.

While your eggs are poaching, melt a smidge more coconut oil in the microwave along with the paprika.

Smear the yoghurt onto your plate. Top with the pile of greens, then make a space and nestle in the poached eggs. Drizzle over the paprika 'butter' and scatter over the almonds. Serve with bread for dipping.

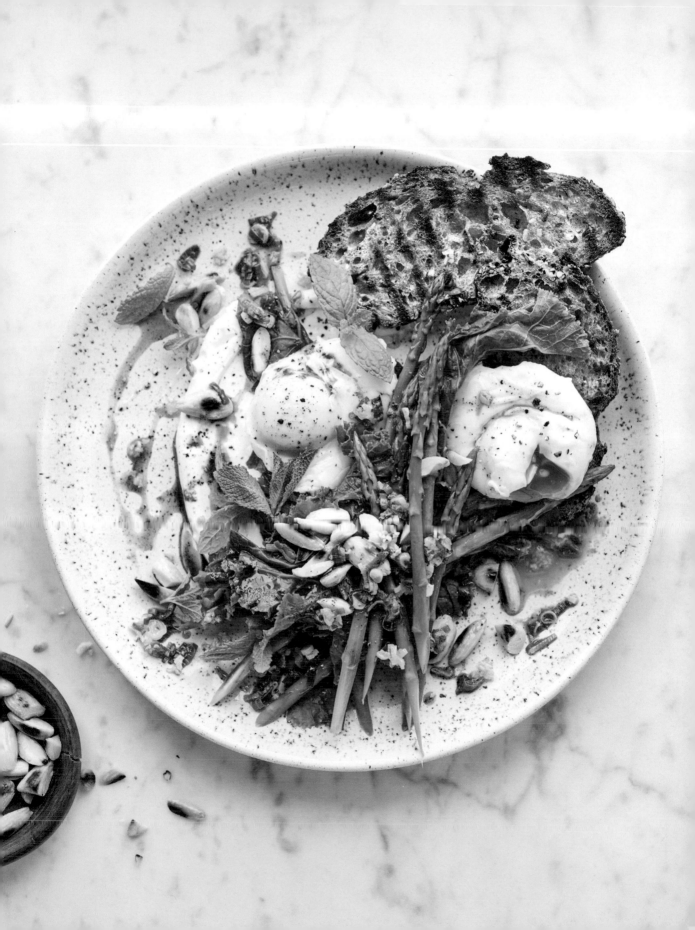

SERVES 1

California scrambled eggs

Ingredients

3 eggs
salt and pepper
1 tbsp coconut oil
½ red chilli – remove the seeds
  if you don't like it hot
8 cherry tomatoes, halved
2 large handfuls of
  spinach leaves
50g feta
½ avocado, de-stoned and sliced
1 tbsp toasted mixed seeds

Method

Crack the eggs into a jug. Whisk well with a fork until the white and yolk combine then season with a generous pinch of salt and pepper.

Melt the coconut oil in a frying pan over a medium heat. Chuck in the chilli and tomatoes. Cook for 2 minutes until the tomatoes have started to burst. Add the spinach and cook until just wilted, then pour in the beaten eggs. Turn down the heat.

Softly scramble the eggs, drawing the cooked eggs from the edges into the middle until the egg is just cooked.

Pile the scrambled eggs onto your plate or serve straight from the pan. Crumble over the feta. Add the sliced avocado alongside, season with a little salt and sprinkle over the mixed seeds.

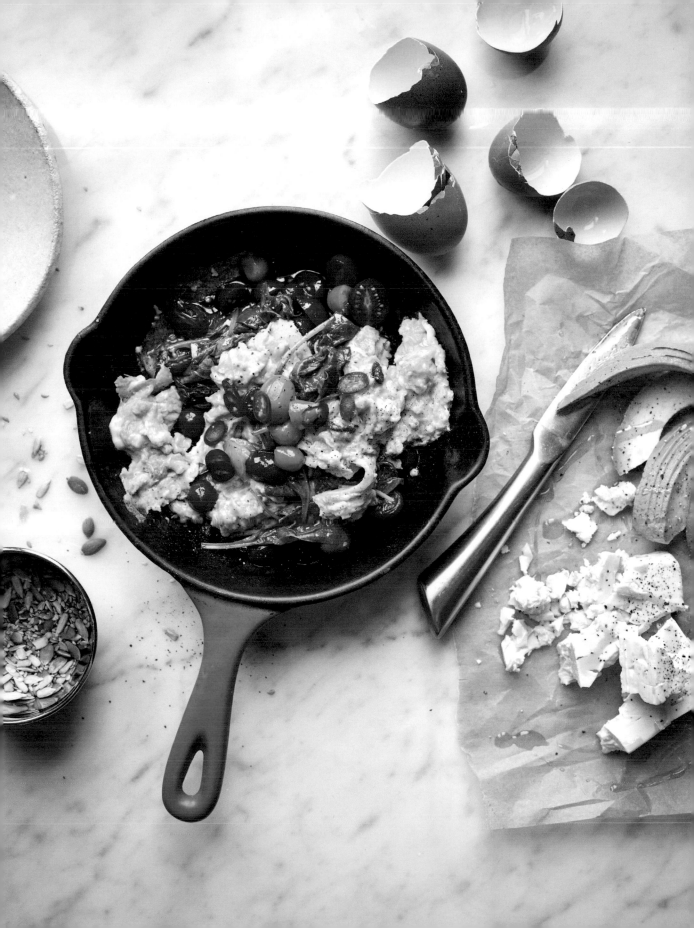

Pimped-up homemade baked beans on toast

LONGER RECIPE
GOOD TO FREEZE
Beans only.

Ingredients

2 tbsp butter
½ red onion, diced
salt and pepper
1 fat clove garlic, finely diced
½ tsp smoked paprika
200g passata
1 x 400g tin of butter or
  cannellini beans, drained
  and rinsed
2 slices of crusty white bread –
  I like sourdough
1 tbsp barbecue sauce
splash of red wine vinegar
1 thick slice of mature cheddar,
  grated – optional

Method

Melt 1 tablespoon of the butter in a saucepan over a low heat. Chuck in the red onion and a good pinch of salt. Cook, stirring regularly for 5 minutes until the onion is softened. Stir in the garlic and smoked paprika and continue cooking for a minute more until everything smells amazing.

Pour in the passata and tip in the beans. Stir everything together then bring to a simmer. Leave to cook for a few minutes until the sauce has thickened while you toast and butter the bread.

Stir the barbecue sauce, splash of vinegar and remaining butter through the beans. Season with salt and pepper, then pile the pimped-up baked beans onto your toast, grating the cheese over the top, if using.

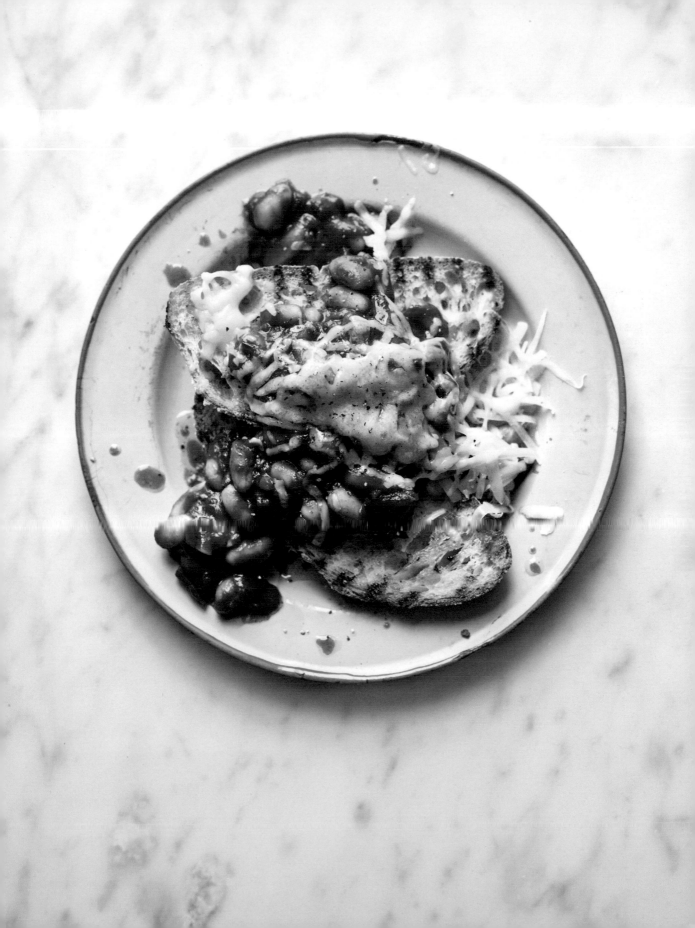

Cheesy French toast with grilled cherry tomatoes and rocket

Ingredients

2 eggs
1 tsp dijon mustard
salt and pepper
40g mature cheddar,
  finely grated
bunch of cherry tomatoes,
  on the vine
1 really thick slice of
  granary bread
1 tbsp coconut oil
large handful of rocket
splash of balsamic vinegar

Method

Preheat your grill to maximum.

Crack the eggs into a shallow bowl that is big enough for dunking in your piece of bread. Whisk the eggs with a fork and add the mustard and a good pinch of salt and pepper. Stir in the grated cheese.

Place the tomatoes on a flat baking sheet and grill for 8 minutes.

While the tomatoes are grilling, dunk your bread into the cheesy egg mix. Leave for about 30 seconds so that the bread soaks up the mix, then flip over and do the same on the other side. Transfer to a plate.

Melt the coconut oil in a frying pan over a medium to high heat. Place the bread in the pan and fry for 2–3 minutes on each side until golden and crisp.

Transfer to a plate, remove the tomatoes from the grill and pile on top with the rocket. Drizzle over the balsamic vinegar. Dream food.

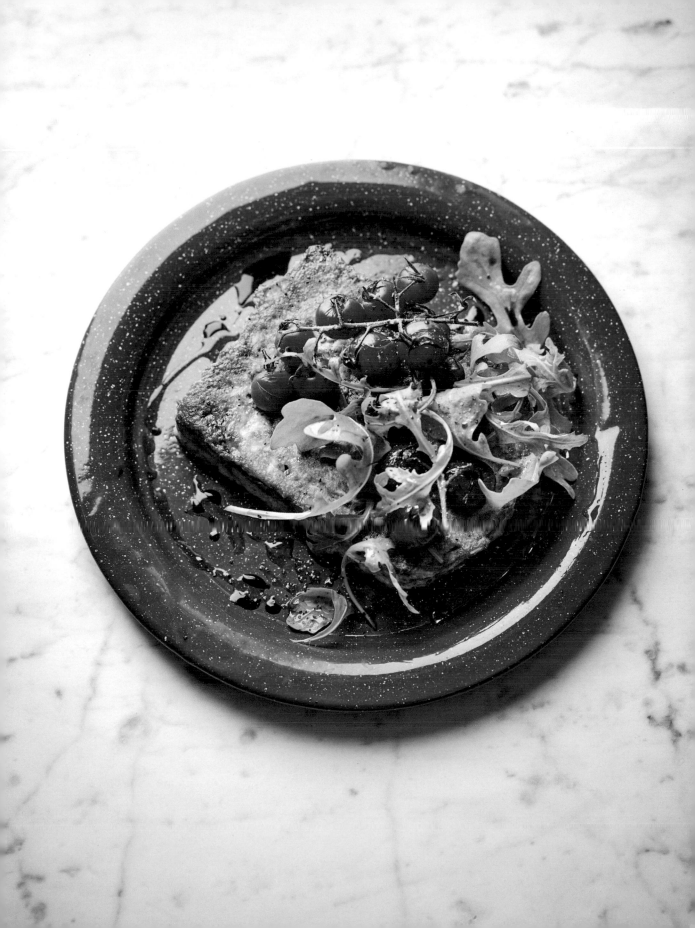

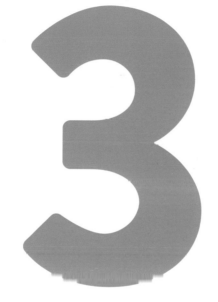

3

'FAST' FOOD

SERVES 1

Chipotle midget tree tacos with sour cream

Ingredients

1 tbsp coconut oil

1 tbsp chipotle paste

200g midget trees (tenderstem broccoli), any bigger stalks sliced in half lengthways

salt

½ red onion, finely sliced

juice of ½ lime, and the rest cut into wedges

pinch of sugar

2 hard-shell tacos

½ avocado, de-stoned and sliced

2 dollops of sour cream

Method

Preheat the oven to 220°C (fan 200°C, gas mark 7). Bring a kettle of water to the boil.

Dollop the coconut oil and chipotle paste onto a baking tray, then scatter over the midget trees. Season with a good pinch of salt and roast in the oven for 14 minutes, turning halfway through.

Place the red onion in a small bowl. While the broccoli is roasting, pour some boiling water from the kettle on top of the onion. Leave for 1 minute, then drain and run the onion under cold water.

Put the onion back in the bowl and squeeze over the lime juice, along with a pinch of salt and the sugar. Leave to lightly pickle.

Assemble your tacos. Fill the tacos with the chipotle midget trees, avocado, sour cream and red onions. Serve with the lime wedges.

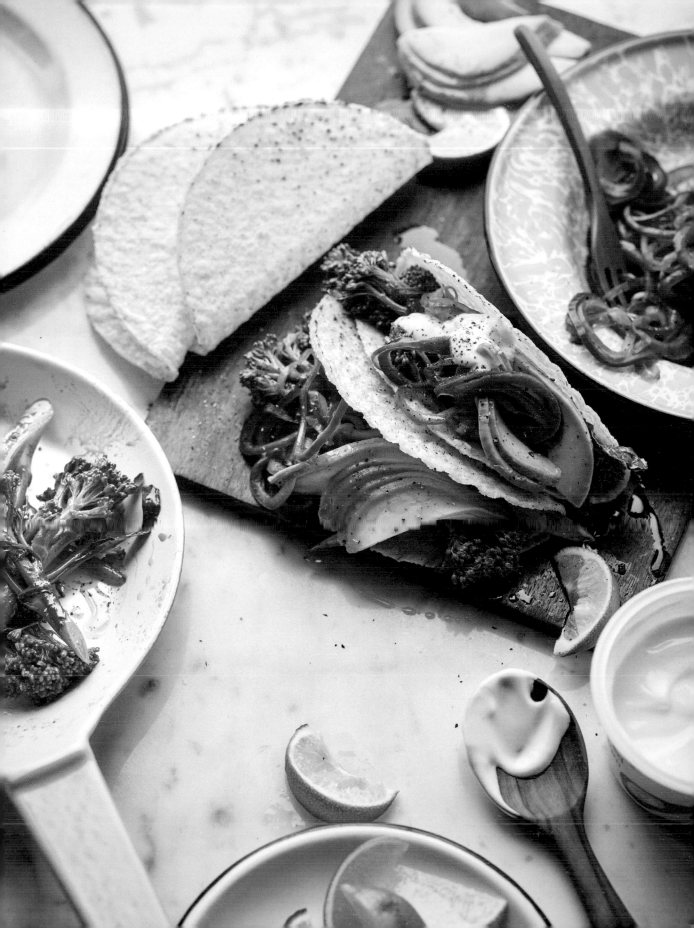

Peri-peri halloumi burger

Ingredients

3 tbsp peri-peri sauce
100g halloumi, cut into
  four slices
1 tbsp mayo
1 baby gem lettuce
1 medium tomato
burger bun

Method

Pour 2 tablespoons of the peri-peri sauce into a shallow bowl. Add the halloumi slices to the bowl and turn them so that both sides are covered in the sauce. Leave to marinate for a few minutes.

While your cheese is marinating, stir the remaining peri-peri into the mayo. Separate the lettuce leaves and slice the tomato into rounds.

Warm a dry non-stick frying pan over a high heat. When it is hot, chuck in the halloumi slices. Dry-fry for 2 minutes on each side, spooning any of the leftover marinade over the cheese as it cooks so that it becomes sticky and crisp. Take off the heat.

Toast your burger bun, then spread the base with the spicy mayo. Stack in the halloumi, lettuce and tomato.

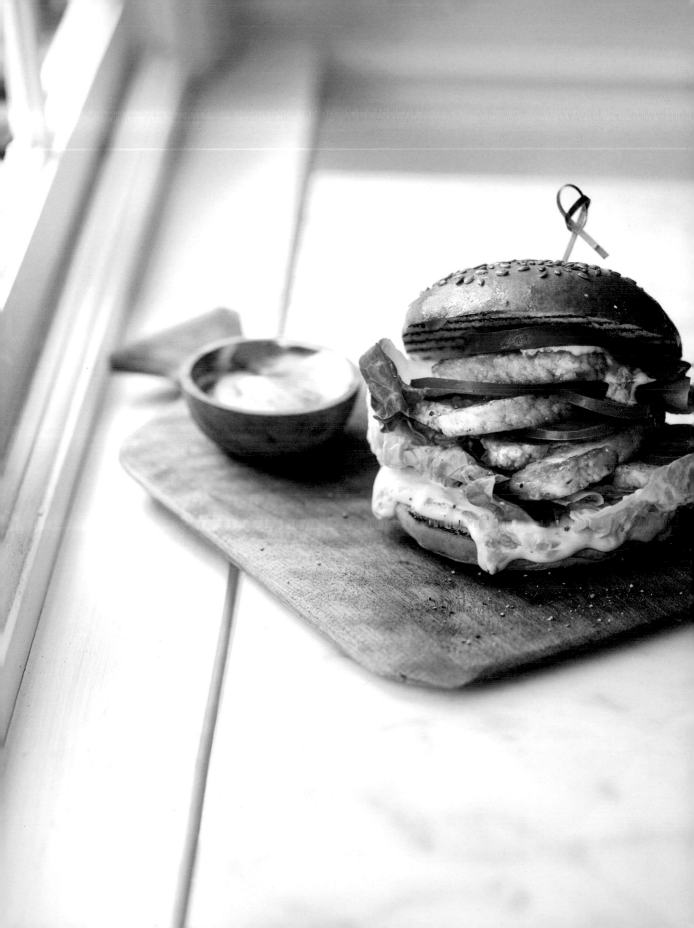

SERVES 1

VE

Satay sweet potato and kale curry

Ingredients

1 sweet potato, peeled and
  chopped into small cubes
1 tbsp coconut oil
½ onion, finely sliced
salt and pepper
1 tsp garlic–ginger paste
pinch of dried chilli flakes,
  plus extra to top
1 tsp tomato puree
1 tsp ground cumin
1½ tbsp peanut butter
big handful of kale, stalks
  removed
juice of 1 lime
spoonful of coconut yoghurt
  and a handful of coriander
  leaves, to serve

Method

Put the sweet potato into a microwaveable bowl, cover with cling film, then zap on high for 8 minutes until soft.

Meanwhile, melt the coconut oil in a saucepan. Slide in the onion with a pinch of salt and cook for 5 minutes until softened. Stir in the garlic–ginger paste, chilli, tomato puree and cumin and cook for 2 minutes more.

Grab your sweet potato from the microwave and tip it into the pan. Give everything a good mix then pour in 400ml boiling water.

Stir in the peanut butter, then use the back of a fork or a potato masher to loosely break up half the sweet potato – this will thicken the curry. Season with salt and pepper.

Let the curry simmer, then stir in the kale. Cook until the kale is just wilted, then take off the heat and squeeze in the lime juice.

Spoon into your bowl then top with the coconut yoghurt, coriander leaves and a few more chilli flakes.

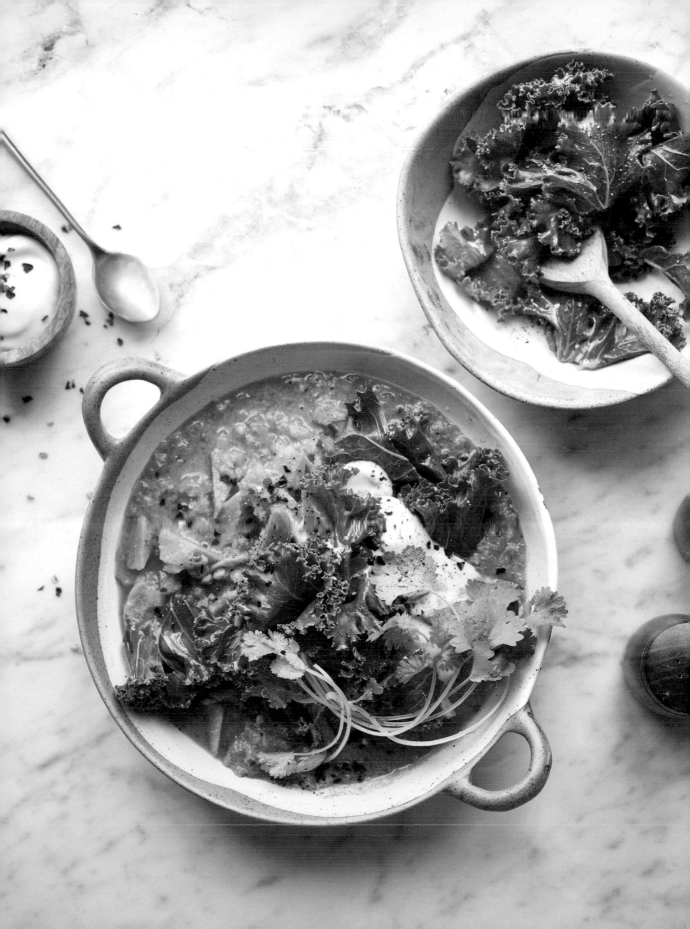

SERVES 1

Homemade baked nachos with fried tomato salsa

Ingredients

2 flour tortillas
2 tbsp olive oil
½ tsp smoked paprika
salt and black pepper
8 cherry tomatoes
½ red onion, finely chopped
1 clove garlic, finely chopped
1 tbsp red wine vinegar
50g pizza mozzarella, grated
50g cheddar, grated
1 tbsp coriander, chopped

Method

Preheat the oven to 200°C (fan 180°C, gas mark 6).

Using kitchen scissors, cut each tortilla into eight triangles, the same size as tortilla crisps. Place them on a baking tray and mix with 1 tablespoon of the olive oil, the paprika and some salt. Spread out into a single layer, then bake for 10 minutes, turning halfway through.

Meanwhile, heat the remaining oil in a frying pan over a high heat. Chuck in the tomatoes and fry for 4 minutes until beginning to blacken and burst. Stir in the red onion and garlic and squash the tomatoes with the back of your spoon so that they roughly break up. Cook for 2 minutes, then remove from the heat and stir through the red wine vinegar along with some salt and pepper.

Scatter the mozzarella and cheddar over the tortilla chips, then bake for a further 5 minutes until the cheese has melted.

Pile the nachos into a bowl, spoon the salsa on top and sprinkle with the coriander.

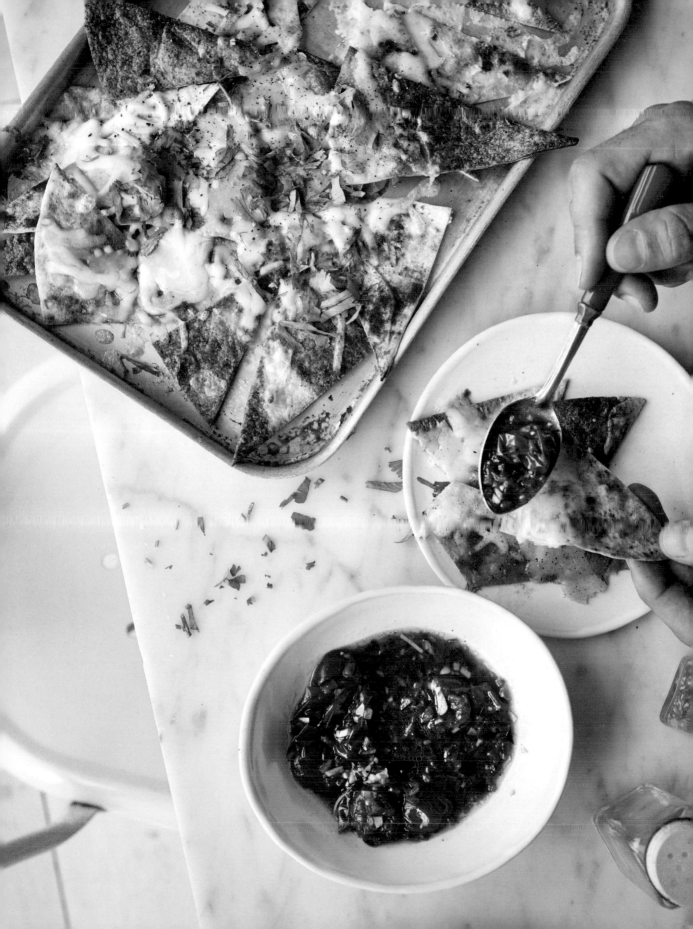

SERVES 1

Tikka masala chickpea fritters with raita

GOOD TO FREEZE
Cooked fritters only.

Ingredients

50g Greek yoghurt
¼ cucumber, grated
handful of mint leaves,
   finely chopped
pinch of ground cumin
salt and pepper
1 x 400g tin of chickpeas,
   drained and rinsed
2 tsp tikka masala curry paste
1 spring onion, halved
1 egg
2 tbsp plain flour
1 tbsp coconut oil
mango chutney, to serve
   – optional

Method

Mix the yoghurt, cucumber, mint, cumin and a pinch of salt and pepper in a bowl. Leave to one side while you make the fritters.

In a small food processor, blitz the chickpeas with the tikka masala curry paste and the spring onion. When finely chopped, crack in the egg and spoon in the flour along with some salt and pepper. Pulse again until everything comes together.

Melt the coconut oil in a frying pan over a medium to high heat. Dollop four spoonfuls of the fritter mix into the pan, using the back of your spoon to flatten slightly. Fry for 2 minutes on each side until golden and warmed through.

Stack the fritters on top of each other on a plate and serve with the raita and mango chutney, if using.

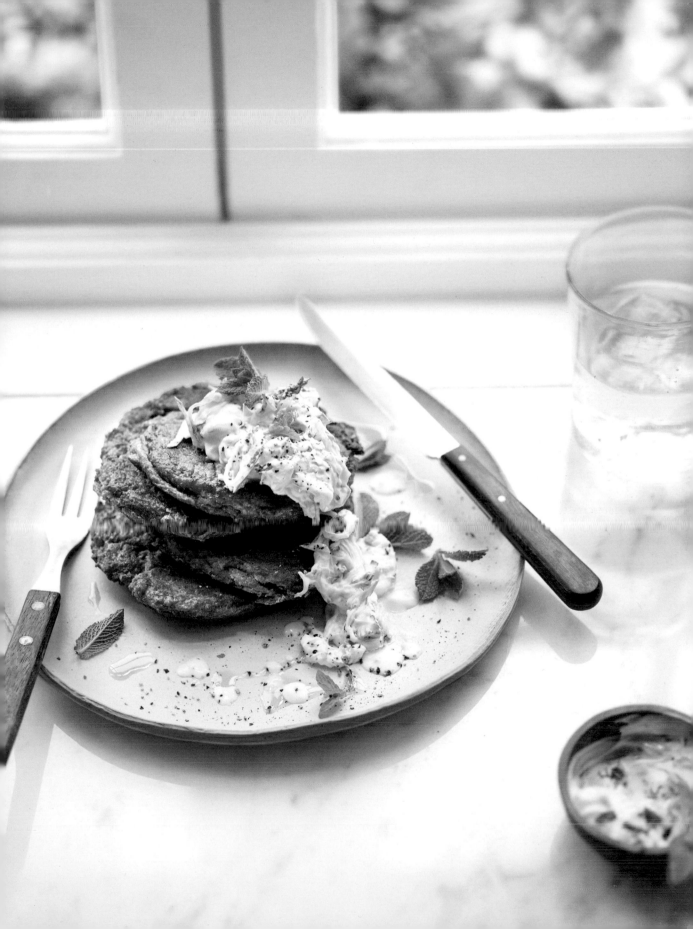

Pak choi and mange tout Pad Thai

Ingredients

100g dried flat rice noodles
juice of 1 lime
2 tbsp soy sauce
1 tsp soft brown sugar
big pinch of dried chilli flakes
1 pak choi
1 fat clove garlic
1 red pepper
1 tbsp coconut oil
100g mange tout
1 egg, beaten
handful of beansprouts
1 tbsp roasted peanuts,
  roughly chopped

Method

Bring a kettle of water to the boil and place the noodles in a heatproof bowl.

Meanwhile, mix together the lime juice, soy sauce, brown sugar and chilli flakes. Leave to one side – this is your Pad Thai sauce.

Pour the boiling water over the noodles and leave for 10 minutes until softened.

Meanwhile, slice the pak choi, garlic and red pepper. Melt the coconut oil in a wok or frying pan over a high heat. Chuck in your pak choi, garlic, pepper and the mange tout. Stir-fry for 2 minutes. Push the veg to one side, then pour in the egg and stir-fry for a minute or so, using your spoon to scramble. Take the pan off the heat for a second.

Drain your noodles and chuck them into the pan along with the Pad Thai sauce and beansprouts. Place the pan back on the heat and cook for 2 minutes until everything is heated through. Top with the peanuts.

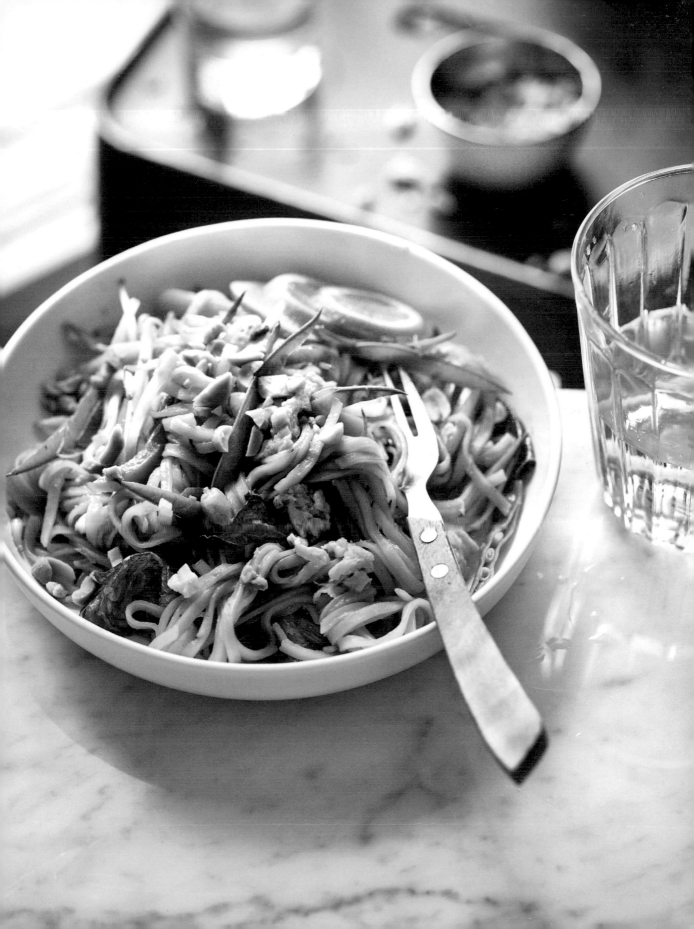

LONGER RECIPE

Ingredients

1 tbsp coconut oil

½ tsp ground turmeric

100g paneer, chopped into
 2cm cubes

½ onion, chopped

salt

1 potato, skin on, cut into
 1cm cubes

½ red chilli, chopped
 – remove the seeds if you
 don't like it hot

1 tsp garlic–ginger paste

1 tsp garam masala

1 tsp cumin seeds

2 large handfuls of baby
 spinach leaves

Paneer
saag aloo

Method

Ping the coconut oil in a small bowl in the microwave.

Pour half the melted oil into a lidded saucepan.

Stir the turmeric into the remaining oil left in the bowl, then add the cubes of paneer and give everything a good stir so that the cheese turns bright yellow. Leave to one side.

Put the saucepan on a medium heat. Add the onion along with a big pinch of salt. Fry for 3 minutes, then chuck in the potato, chilli, garlic–ginger paste, garam masala and cumin seeds. Cook, stirring, for 3 minutes.

Pour 150ml water into the pan, cover with the lid and cook for 8 minutes, stirring occasionally.

Meanwhile, place a non-stick frying pan over a medium to high heat. Add the paneer along with the oil and turmeric, then fry for 2 minutes on each side until crisp and golden. Turn down the heat to the lowest it can go and leave the cheese in the pan to keep warm.

Check the potatoes are cooked through by prodding them with a knife. Chuck in the spinach, and when wilted, spoon the saag aloo into a bowl and top with the crisp paneer.

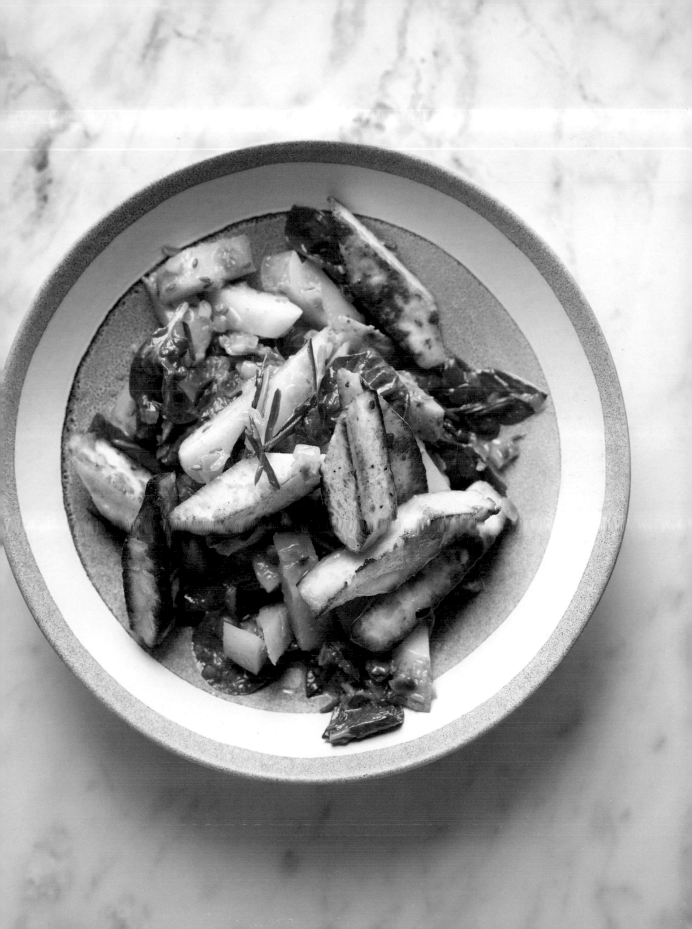

SERVES 1

VE

Cheeky Chinese tofu with sesame greens

Ingredients

150g firm tofu, drained and
  chopped into 2cm cubes
1 tbsp soy sauce
2 tbsp hoisin sauce
1 tbsp rice wine vinegar
1 clove garlic
1 tbsp sesame oil
100g sugarsnap peas
3 large handfuls of kale,
  stalks removed
salt
1 tsp sesame seeds
rice, to serve

Method

Preheat your grill to maximum.

Line a baking tray with tin foil, then put the tofu on top.

Mix together the soy sauce, 1 tablespoon of the hoisin sauce and the rice wine vinegar. Crush in the garlic, stir, then pour the sauce over the tofu. Give everything a good toss so that the tofu is completely covered in the sauce, then spread out the pieces in a single layer.

Grill the tofu for 8 minutes, turning halfway and spooning the sauce over the tofu.

Meanwhile, pour the sesame oil into a frying pan over a high heat. Chuck in the sugarsnap peas, kale and 1 tablespoon of water. Fry until the kale has wilted and the peas are tender. Season with salt.

Transfer the greens to a plate, then sprinkle over the sesame seeds. Serve the tofu alongside the steaming sesame veg. Drizzle over the remaining hoisin sauce and serve with rice.

SERVES 1

Tikka masala cauliflower naan pizza

Ingredients

1 tbsp coconut oil
½ head of small cauliflower, florets only
1 tbsp tikka masala curry paste
salt and pepper
½ green chilli, finely sliced – optional
1 naan bread
2 tbsp natural yoghurt
dollop of mango chutney
a few coriander leaves
1 tbsp toasted flaked almonds

Method

Preheat the oven to 220°C (fan 200°C, gas mark 7). Dollop the coconut oil into a high-sided roasting tin and transfer to the oven to heat up.

Meanwhile, put the cauliflower florets into a large microwaveable bowl with 1 tablespoon of water. Cover with cling film and zap on high for 1 minute.

Remove the cling film, then stir through the tikka masala curry paste along with some salt and pepper.

Carefully bring the hot roasting tin out of the oven. Slide in the curried cauliflower and spread out into a single layer. Roast in the oven for 12 minutes.

While the cauliflower is roasting, finely slice the green chilli, if using.

Wrap the naan in tin foil and place in the bottom of the oven for the final 4 minutes of the cauliflower's cooking time.

Unwrap the naan and place it on your plate. Spread over the yoghurt for the 'pizza sauce' then spoon over the tikka masala cauliflower. Dot over the mango chutney, then scatter over the green chilli, coriander and flaked almonds.

Huevos rancheros bagel

Ingredients

1 tbsp coconut oil
1 tsp chipotle paste
200g black beans, drained
  and rinsed
salt and pepper
juice of ½ lime
1 tbsp coriander, chopped
1 egg
1 bagel, sliced in half
½ avocado, de-stoned and sliced
50g feta, crumbled
drizzle of hot sauce, such as
  Sriracha, to serve – optional

Method

Melt half the coconut oil in a frying pan over a medium heat. Stir in the chipotle paste, then tip in the black beans along with some salt and pepper. Use the back of your spoon to roughly mash some of the beans. Tip into a bowl, then stir through the lime juice and chopped coriander.

Put the pan back on the heat (don't bother washing it – extra flavour). Melt the remaining coconut oil then crack in your egg and fry to your liking.

While the egg is frying, toast the bagel.

Assemble your huevos rancheros bagel. Smoosh the beans onto the bottom of the bagel, lay over the sliced avocado then top with the fried egg. Crumble over the feta and drizzle with hot sauce, if using.

Top with the other bagel half and enjoy.

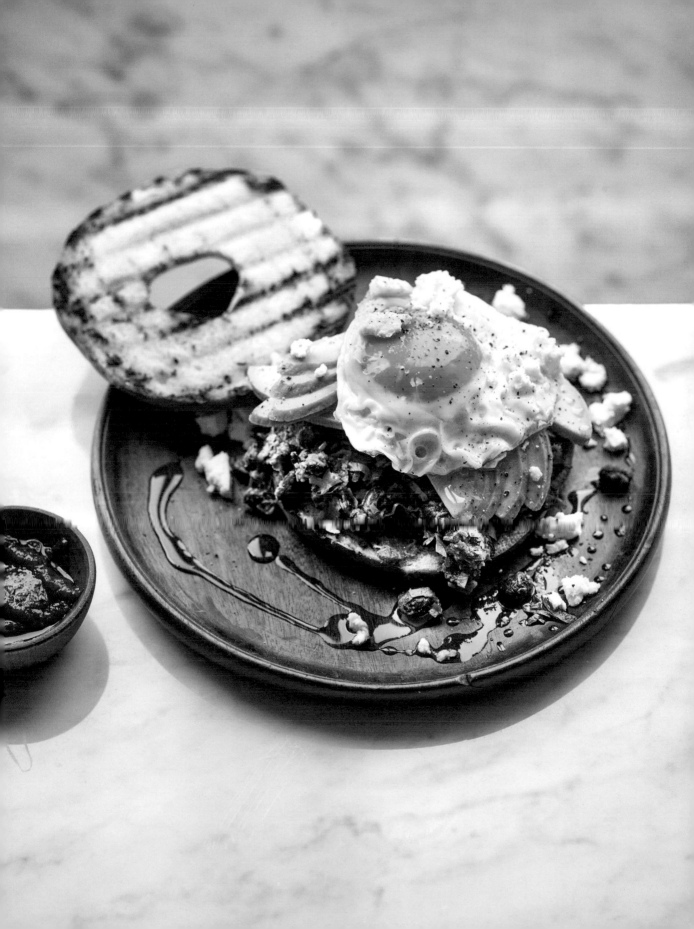

Teriyaki tofu with midget trees and noodles

Ingredients

100g firm tofu, drained and
    chopped into 2cm cubes
2 tbsp teriyaki sauce
1 tbsp coconut oil
1 tsp garlic–ginger paste
2 spring onions, finely sliced
6 midget trees (tenderstem
    broccoli), each cut into
    three pieces
6 baby sweetcorn, sliced in
    half lengthways
150g 'straight to wok'
    egg noodles
30g cashews, roughly chopped
handful of coriander,
    roughly chopped, plus
    a few sprigs to serve
1 tbsp soy sauce

Method

Pat the tofu cubes dry with a square of kitchen roll.
Mix the teriyaki sauce with 1 tablespoon of water.

Melt half the coconut oil in a frying pan over a high heat.
Add in the cubes of tofu to the pan and fry for 4 minutes,
turning the tofu regularly so it crisps evenly. Spoon in
two-thirds of the teriyaki sauce, tossing everything together
so that each piece gets nice and sticky, then turn down the
heat to its lowest to keep the tofu warm.

Meanwhile, melt the remaining coconut oil in a frying
pan over a high heat. Stir in the garlic–ginger paste,
spring onions, midget trees and baby sweetcorn. Fry for
4 minutes.

Chuck in the noodles, chopped cashews, coriander,
soy sauce and remaining teriyaki sauce. Give everything
a good stir and cook for 1–2 minutes, or until the noodles
are heated through.

Pile the noodles into a bowl and top with the teriyaki tofu.
Scatter over a little coriander to serve.

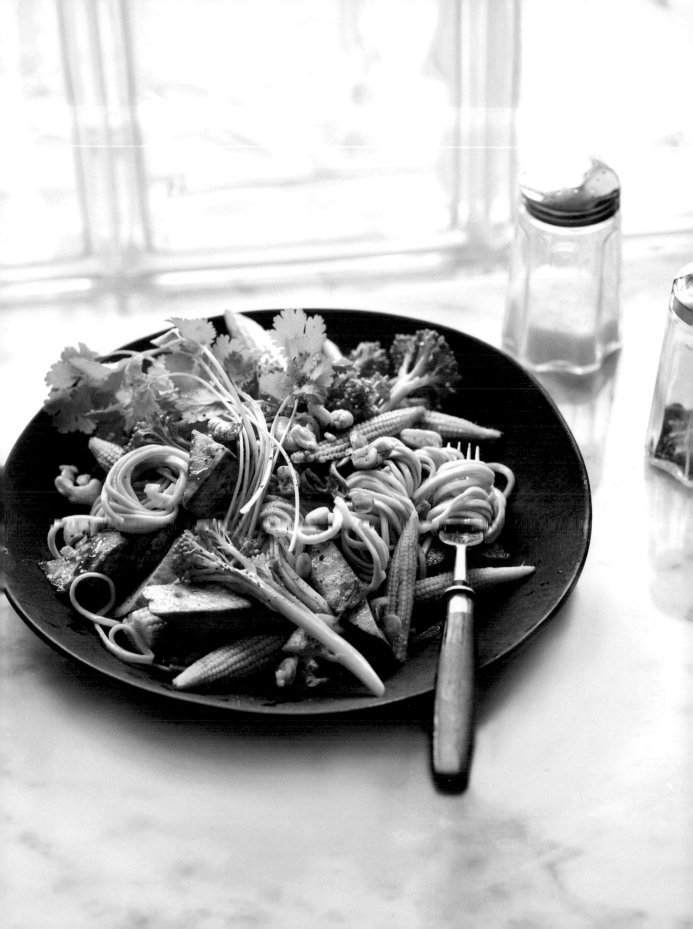

SERVES 1

Ingredients

¼ cucumber
½ tbsp white wine vinegar
salt and pepper
150g falafel
1 tbsp tahini
50g Greek yoghurt
juice of ½ lemon
⅙ red cabbage
1 large tortilla wrap
1 tsp toasted sesame seeds
olive oil, for drizzling – optional

Sesame falafel wrap

Method

Preheat the oven to 200°C (fan 180°C/gas mark 6).

While the oven is heating, slice the cucumber in half lengthways and use a spoon to scoop out the seeds, then cut into half-moon pieces. Put the cucumber into a bowl and pour over the white wine vinegar along with a pinch of salt. Give everything a good stir, then leave to pickle.

Put your falafel on a baking tray. Reheat in the oven according to packet instructions, around 8 minutes.

Meanwhile, mix together the tahini, Greek yoghurt and some salt and pepper. Squeeze in the lemon juice, adding as much as you want to taste and a splash of water to get it to a thick drizzling consistency.

Use the coarse side of the grater to shred the red cabbage into a bowl. Mix half the tahini yoghurt through the red cabbage in the bowl.

Either griddle the tortilla on both sides or cover it with tin foil, then place in the oven briefly to heat up. Spread the remaining tahini yoghurt down the centre, then scatter over the red cabbage mix and pickled cucumber. Top with the falafel then sprinkle over the sesame seeds and drizzle with olive oil, if liked. Winning.

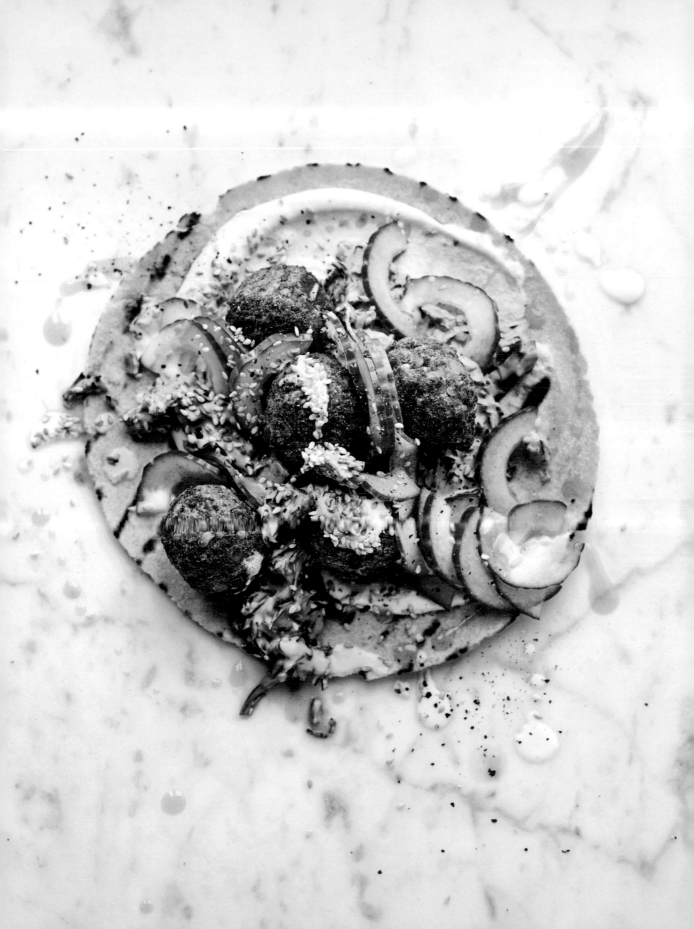

Joe's ultimate pizza

LONGER RECIPE

Ingredients

olive oil
1 clove garlic, crushed
big pinch of dried chilli flakes
200g passata
salt and pepper
2 flour tortillas, wholemeal
  or white is fine
½ ball of mozzarella, torn (75g)
4 pitted green olives, halved
1 egg
large handful of rocket

Method

Preheat the oven to 200°C (fan 180°C, gas mark 6). Lightly grease a flat baking sheet with olive oil.

Stir the crushed garlic, chilli flakes and passata together. Season with salt and pepper.

Place a tortilla on the greased baking sheet. Spread over a spoonful of the seasoned passata, then stick the second tortilla on the top.

Spread over the rest of the passata, then scatter over the mozzarella and olive halves. Slide your baking sheet into the oven, then pull the rack out slightly, and with the door ajar, crack the egg into the middle of the pizza. Slide the rack back in, push the door shut and cook for 10 minutes until the tortilla base is crisp, the white of the egg is set but the yolk remains jammy.

Take your tortilla pizza out the oven, scatter with the rocket and drizzle with a little olive oil.

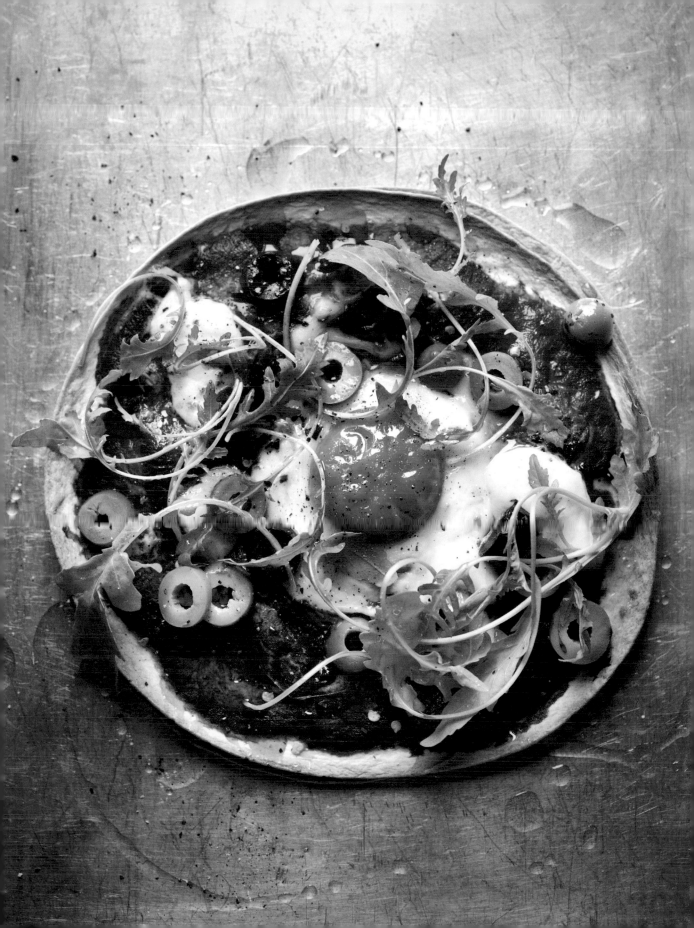

SERVES 1

MAKE AHEAD
Reheat in the microwave.

Ingredients

½ small butternut squash,
  peeled and chopped
½ avocado, de-stoned
2 spring onions, finely sliced
  (green bits and all)
juice of 1 lime
salt and pepper
½ tbsp coconut oil
1 clove garlic, finely sliced
½ x 400g tin of black beans,
  drained and rinsed
1 tbsp barbecue fajita seasoning
2 flour tortillas
30g cheddar
2 drizzles of barbecue sauce

Barbecue butternut quesadilla

Method

Put the butternut squash in a large microwaveable bowl with 1 tablespoon of water. Cover with cling film, then zap on high for 8 minutes until cooked.

Scoop out the avocado and place in a small bowl with half the spring onion and half the lime juice. Roughly mash with a fork and season with salt and pepper.

Melt the coconut oil in a large frying pan over a medium heat. Add the remaining spring onion and the garlic. Fry for 1 minute, then tip in the black beans and fajita seasoning. Give everything a good stir and cook for 2 minutes more.

Tip the bean mixture into the butternut squash bowl, which by now will be cooked. Roughly mash everything together with a fork. Squeeze in the remaining lime juice and season with salt and pepper.

Put the pan back on a high heat (don't bother washing it – extra flavour). Place the first tortilla in the pan and pile the butternut and black bean mixture on top.

Grate over the cheddar, then drizzle with a little barbecue sauce and put the other tortilla on top. Chop into pieces and chow down with the avo dip.

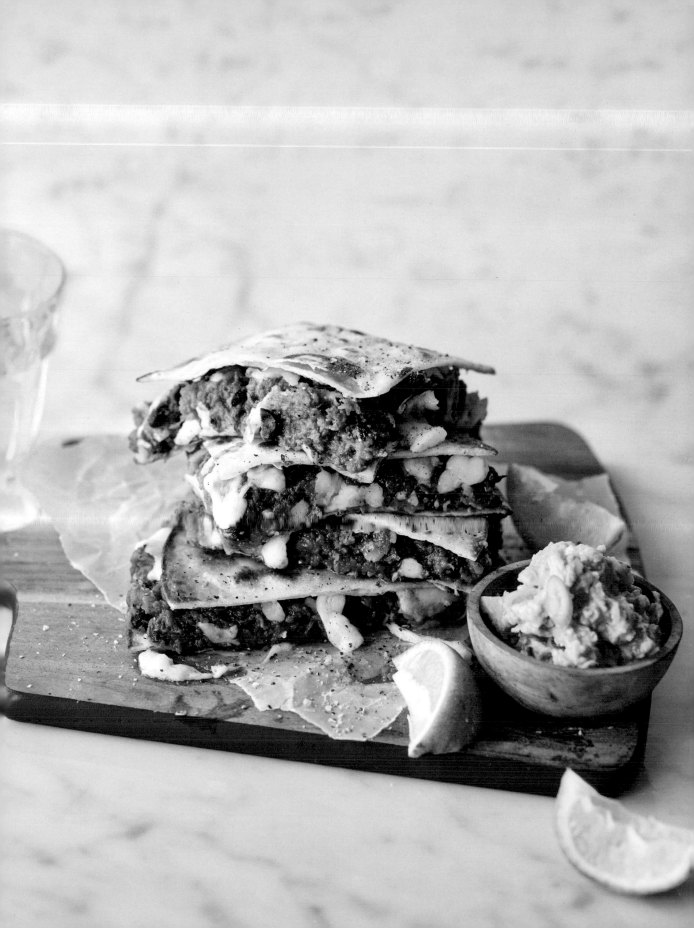

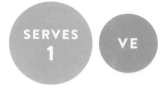

SERVES
1

VE

MAKE AHEAD
GOOD TO FREEZE

Ingredients

½ tsp coconut oil

2 tbsp Thai red curry paste
– make sure it is vegan

small piece of ginger, finely
chopped

1 x 200ml tin of coconut cream

200ml veg stock (from a cube
is fine)

100g mange tout

100g baby sweetcorn, halved
lengthways

100g 'straight to wok' rice
noodles

juice of 1 lime

handful of coriander leaves

2 tbsp toasted cashews

Baby sweetcorn and mange tout laksa

Method

Melt the coconut oil in a saucepan over a medium heat. Stir in the Thai red curry paste and ginger. Cook for 1 minute until it smells fragrant. Pour in the coconut cream and veg stock.

Bring to the boil, then drop in the mange tout and baby sweetcorn. Simmer for 3 minutes until the veg is nearly tender, then chuck in the rice noodles and cook for 1 minute more. Squeeze in the lime juice.

Ladle into your bowl. Top with the coriander leaves and toasted cashews.

JOE'S
TOP TIP

If you can't get hold of fresh rice noodles, use dried and soak them in boiling water while you make the laksa, then drain and add them in at the end.

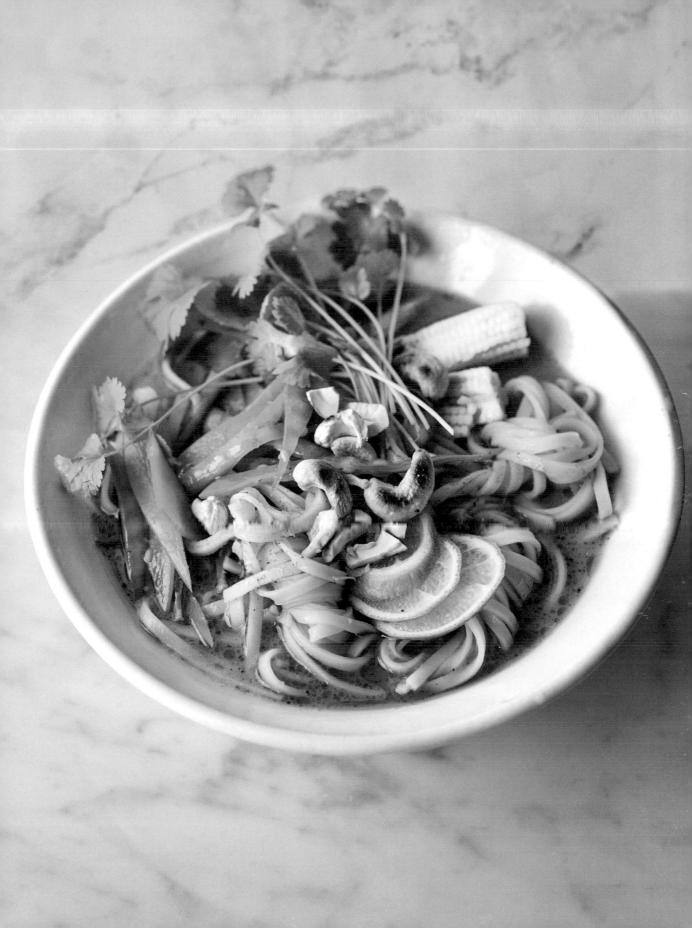

Joe's ultimate veggie burger

Ingredients

50g cashews

2 tbsp olive oil

1 onion, finely chopped

2 portobello mushrooms, cut
  into cubes

2 cloves garlic, finely chopped

salt and pepper

125g (about ½ pack)
  pre-cooked mixed grains

1 x 400g tin of kidney beans,
  drained and rinsed

2 tsp Marmite

1 tsp smoked paprika

1 egg yolk

100g mature cheddar,
  finely grated

4 burger buns, sliced in half

drizzle of ketchup, mayo and/or
  mustard, to serve

2 baby gem lettuce, leaves
  separated, to serve

handful of gherkins, sliced in
  half, to serve – optional

Method

Tip the cashews into a dry, very large frying pan and toast over a medium heat until lightly browned and smelling nutty.

Put the pan back on the heat and pour in 1 tablespoon of the olive oil. Chuck in the onion, mushrooms and garlic along with some salt and pepper. Cook for 10 minutes until everything is soft and all the water from the mushrooms has evaporated. Add the mixed grains to the pan and use the back of your spoon to break up the pieces. Stir well to combine, then take off the heat.

Tip half of this mushroom mixture into a food processor along with all of the cashew nuts and the kidney beans. Blitz until smooth.

Scrape into a large bowl and add the remaining whole mushroom mix, Marmite, smoked paprika, egg yolk and half the grated cheese. Beat well with a wooden spoon until everything is completely combined, then season with a generous amount of salt and pepper.

Wipe out the frying pan. Pour in the remaining olive oil and place over a medium heat. Shape the burgers into four patties straight into the pan. Fry for 3 minutes on one side until browned and crisp. Carefully flip over and cook on the other side for 2 minutes. Place a pile of the remaining cheese over the burgers. Put a lid on the pan and cook for 1 minute or so until melted.

Toast your burger buns, and drizzle with some ketchup/mayo and mustard. Stack in the burger and top with the lettuce and some gherkins, if using.

JOE'S TOP TIP Be careful when you are flipping over the burgers as they are a little soft – but no one likes a dry, stodgy veggie burger!

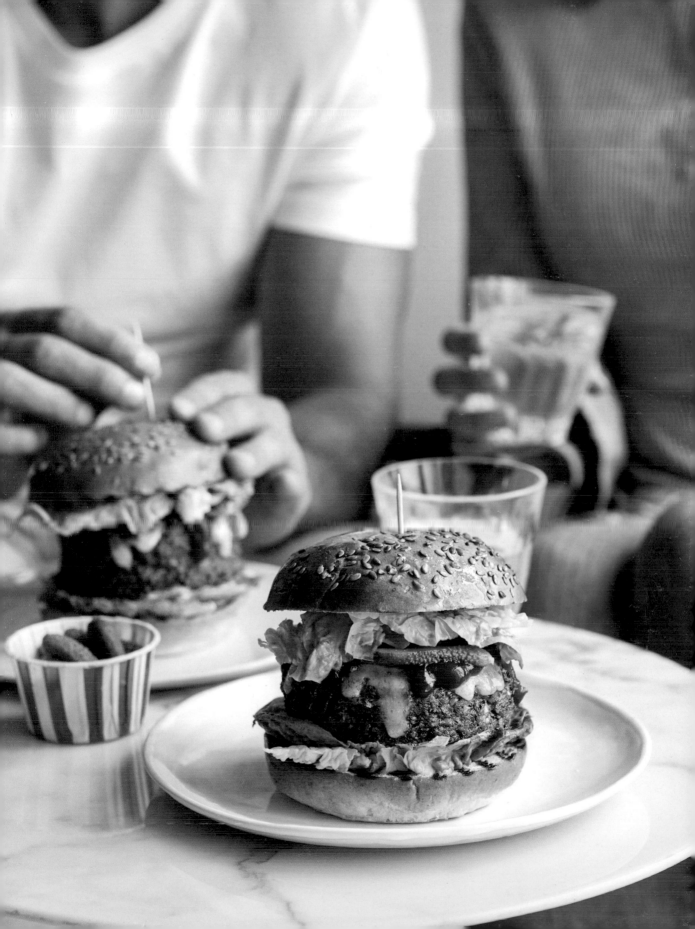

Joe's midget tree and cheddar tots

Ingredients

smidge of melted coconut oil,
  for greasing
1 large midget tree (broccoli
  head)
60g mature cheddar cheese,
  grated
½ onion, finely chopped
handful of parsley, chopped
60g breadcrumbs
1 egg
salt and black pepper
2 handfuls of rocket
1 yellow pepper, sliced
squeeze of lemon juice
ketchup, to serve

Method

Preheat the oven to 200°C (fan 180°C, gas mark 6). Bring a kettle of water to the boil and brush a baking tray with the coconut oil.

Pour enough boiling water into a saucepan to fill it halfway and place over a medium heat. Put your large midget tree (broccoli head) into the water, leafy side down. Whack a lid on the pan (chop the end of the stalk off if you can't fit the lid on) and steam for 2–4 minutes, until just soft. Drain and re-fill the pan with cold water, to cool down the broccoli and halt the cooking. When cold, shake off all the water and chop it finely.

Put the chopped broccoli, grated cheese, onion, parsley, breadcrumbs and egg into a bowl. Season with salt and pepper, then use your hands to work it all together. Roll into 12–14 tots and place them onto the oiled tray. Bake at the top of the oven for 15 minutes until golden brown.

While the tots are baking, toss the rocket and yellow pepper together with the lemon juice. Season to taste with more salt and pepper.

Pile the tots on a plate, put the salad on one side and serve with ketchup.

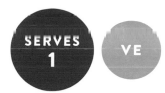

SERVES 1   **VE**

MAKE AHEAD
GOOD TO FREEZE

Ingredients

1 tbsp coconut oil

2 spring onions, finely sliced

1 small aubergine, diced
 as small as possible

2 tbsp Thai green curry paste
 (but check the packet to make
 sure it is vegan)

1 lemongrass stalk, bashed

1 x 200ml tin of coconut cream

pinch of sugar

handful of green beans, halved

1 tsp soy sauce

½ lime

handful of basil leaves

1 tbsp toasted cashew nuts

rice, to serve

Thai green aubergine curry

Method

Melt the coconut oil in a saucepan over a medium heat. Add the spring onions. Fry for 2 minutes until softened. Chuck in the aubergine and give everything a good mix. Fry for 4 minutes until beginning to soften.

Stir in the curry paste and lemongrass. Cook for 1 minute until it smells fragrant, then spoon in the coconut cream. Re-fill the can with water and pour that into the saucepan. Stir in a pinch of sugar, then turn up the heat and leave the curry to cook for 5 minutes.

Chuck in the green beans. Cook for 3–4 minutes until the beans and aubergine are cooked.

Remove the curry from the heat, season with the soy sauce and lime juice. Cut any remaining lime into a wedge for serving.

Spoon the curry into a bowl, removing the lemongrass stalk. Scatter over the basil leaves and toasted cashew nuts. Serve with the lime wedge and rice.

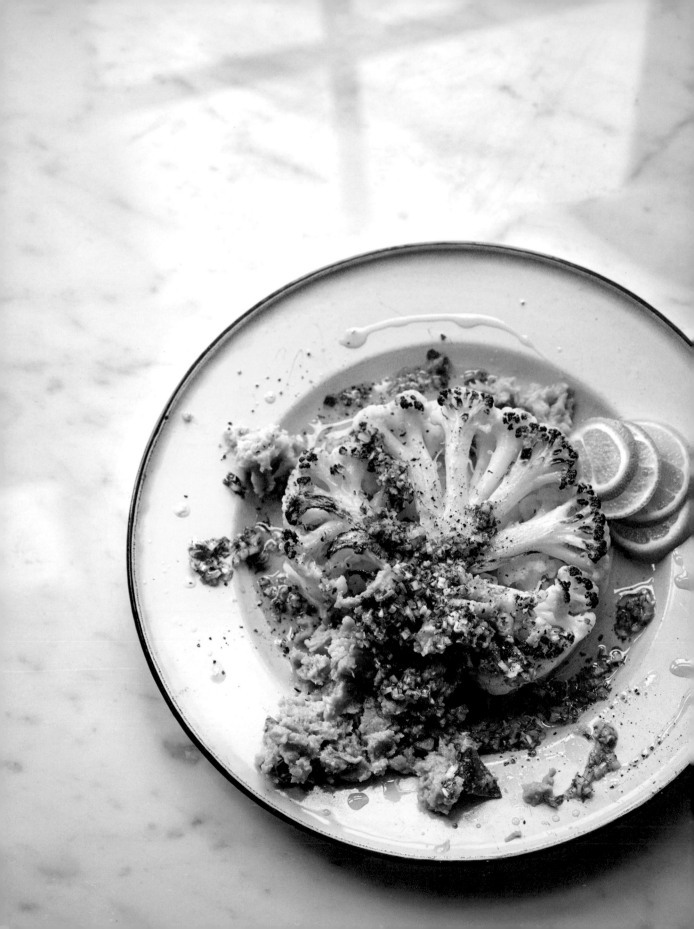

SERVES 1 **VE**

Cauliflower steak with cheat's chimichurri

Ingredients

1 sweet potato, skin on
½ lime, cut into wedges
1 cauliflower steak (1 x 1–2cm
  slice lengthways through
  the centre of a head of
  cauliflower)
1 small clove garlic
2½ tbsp olive oil
1 small shallot, finely chopped
1 tbsp parsley, finely chopped
big pinch of dried oregano
salt and pepper
splash of red wine vinegar

Method

Cut the sweet potato into smallish cubes. Place in a microwaveable bowl with the lime wedges, cover with cling film, then zap on high for 10 minutes until completely cooked.

While the sweet potato is cooking, place the cauliflower steak in a lidded frying pan. Pour in 50ml water and put the lid on, then cook over a high heat for 7 minutes until all the water has evaporated.

Meanwhile, make the cheat's chimichurri sauce by crushing the garlic clove into 1½ tablespoons of the olive oil. Mix in the shallot, parsley and dried oregano. Stir, then add salt, pepper and the red wine vinegar to taste.

Come back to the cauliflower. Take off the lid and flip the cauliflower steak. Pour in the remaining olive oil. Season and cook without the lid for 5 minutes.

Remove the lime wedges from the cooked sweet potato, squeezing out any juice. Season with salt and pepper, then mash in the bowl with a fork. Spoon onto a plate. Top with the cauliflower steak, browned side up, and drizzle over the chimichurri sauce.

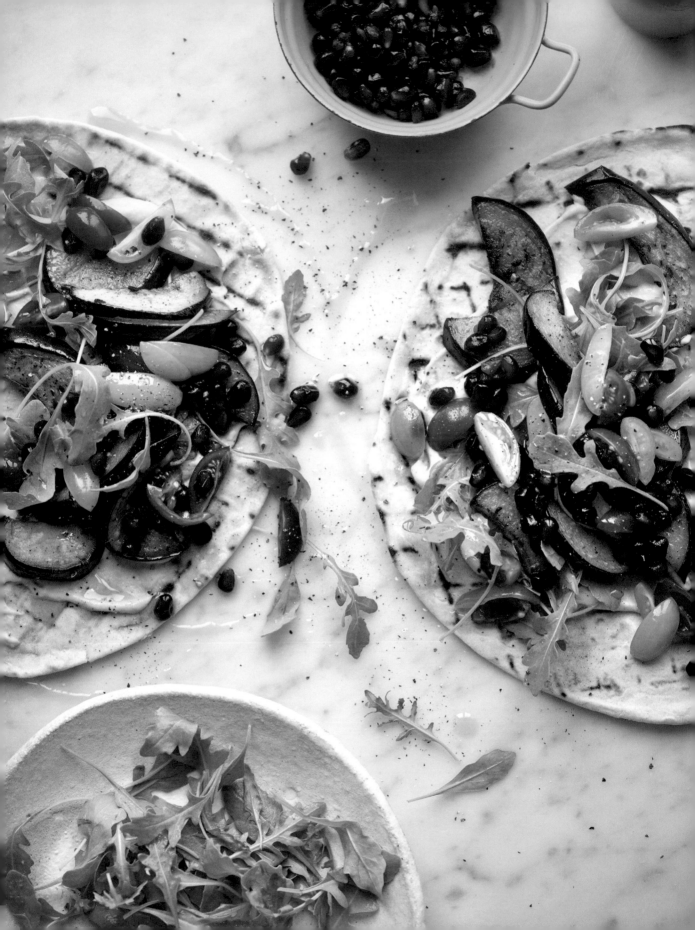

SERVES
1

VE

Fried aubergine, pomegranate and hummus flatbreads

Ingredients

5 cherry tomatoes – I like a
   mix of yellow and red
1 tbsp pomegranate seeds
½ tbsp red wine or sherry
   vinegar
salt and pepper
1 tbsp coconut oil
½ tsp ground cumin
¼ tsp chilli powder
½ aubergine, thinly sliced into
   half-moons
1 large flatbread
3 tbsp hummus
handful of rocket

Method

Roughly chop the cherry tomatoes then scrape them into a bowl with the juices. Stir in the pomegranate seeds, red wine vinegar and a good pinch of salt and pepper. Set aside.

Zap the coconut oil in a large bowl in the microwave for 30 seconds until melted. Stir in the ground cumin and chilli powder along with a pinch of salt and pepper. Chuck in the aubergine then use your hands to coat all of the slices in the oil and spice mix.

Put a large non-stick frying pan over a medium heat. Lay the aubergine slices in the pan, trying to get all of them in a single layer. Fry for 5 minutes on each side until golden and crisp on the outside and squidgy on the inside.

Take the pan off the heat. Zap your flatbread in the microwave to warm it then spread with the hummus. Spoon over the tomato–pomegranate salsa, then pile the aubergine slices on top. Mix the rocket with any remaining vinegar left in the bottom of the tomato bowl, then scatter that into your flatbread. Roll up and gobble down.

JOE'S
TOP TIP

Mixing tomatoes with red wine or sherry vinegar helps to intensify their flavour.

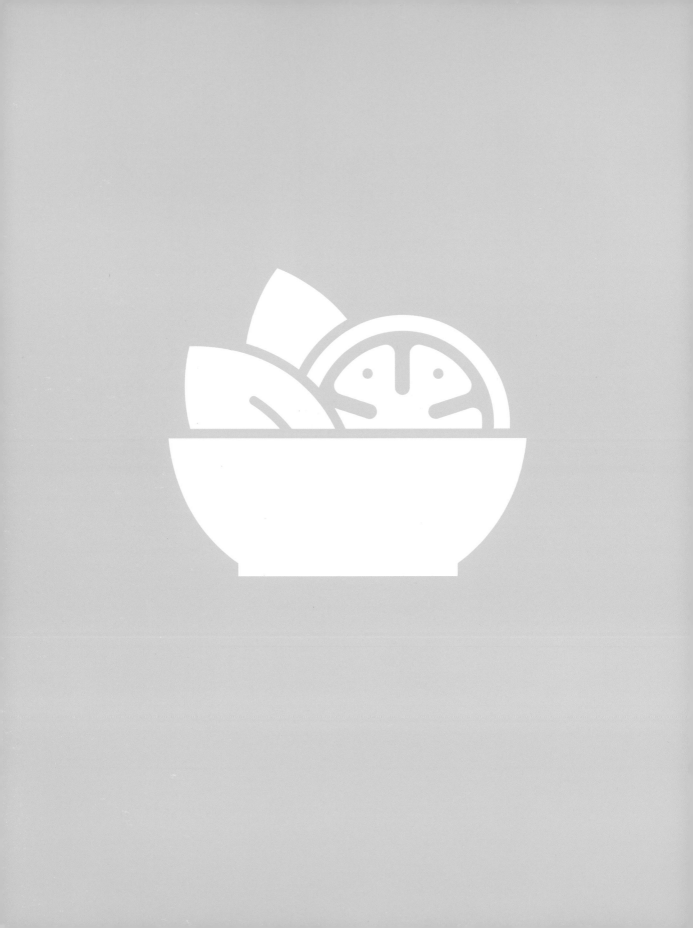

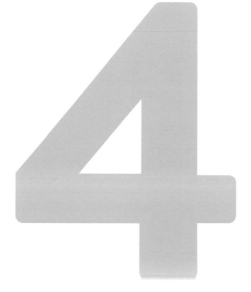

4

HOT AND COLD SALADS

SERVES 1

Charred sprout, feta and pomegranate salad

Ingredients

200g Brussels sprouts, trimmed and halved
2 tbsp coconut oil
½ red onion, finely sliced
2 tbsp pomegranate seeds
pinch of dried chilli flakes
salt
1½ tbsp balsamic vinegar
6 radishes, roughly chopped
handful of parsley, roughly chopped
juice of ½ lemon
50g feta
2 tbsp toasted pumpkin seeds

Method

Put the sprouts in a microwaveable bowl with 1 tablespoon of water. Cover with cling film and zap on high for 1 minute, then drain off the water.

Melt the coconut oil in a large frying pan over a medium heat. Place in the sprouts, cut-side down, in a single layer in the pan and leave to cook for 10 minutes without turning.

While the sprouts are cooking, chuck the red onion, pomegranate seeds, chilli flakes and a pinch of salt into a small bowl. Pour in the vinegar and give everything a good mix to combine, then set aside – this will lightly pickle the onions.

Go back to your sprouts, which after 10 minutes will be nearly tender. Turn the heat up to high and pour the vinegar from the onions into the pan. Bubble away for 2 minutes so that the sprouts get sticky and caramelized.

Take the pan off the heat, then stir in the onion mixture, radishes, parsley and lemon juice.

Pile the charred sprout salad on your plate, crumble the feta on top and scatter with pumpkin seeds.

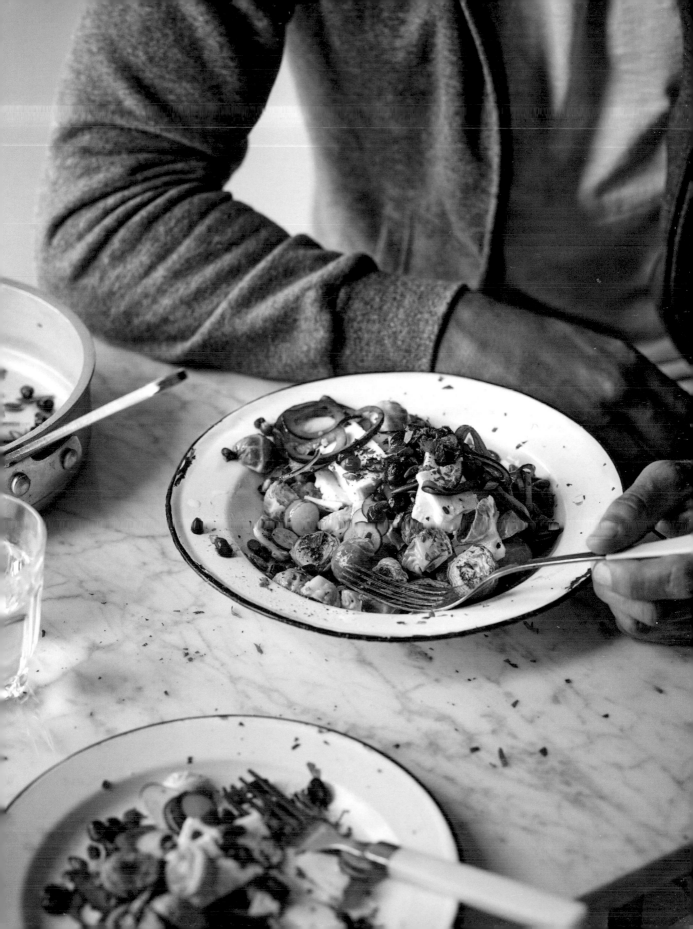

Curried carrot and mixed grains with coriander yoghurt dressing

MAKE AHEAD
Keep the dressing separate.

Ingredients

1 tbsp coconut oil

3 medium carrots, peeled and roughly chopped

½ tbsp curry powder

salt and pepper

50g Greek yoghurt

small bunch of coriander (stalks and all), roughly chopped

½ green chilli, de-seeded and roughly chopped

juice of ½ lime

small knob of ginger

30g toasted almonds, roughly chopped

1 x 250g pack pre-cooked mixed grains

Method

Preheat the oven to 220°C (fan 200°C, gas mark 7). Dollop the coconut oil into a high-sided roasting tin then place it in the oven to heat up.

Meanwhile, put the carrots into a large microwaveable bowl with 1 tablespoon of water. Cover with cling film and zap on high for 2 minutes.

Carefully bring the hot roasting tin out of the oven. Tip in the carrots and sprinkle with the curry powder and some salt and pepper. Mix everything together with a couple of spoons or some tongs, then separate the carrots into a single layer. Roast in the oven for 12 minutes.

While the carrots are roasting, make the dressing. Put the yoghurt, coriander, green chilli and lime juice into a small food processor. Grate in the ginger and blitz until smooth. Season with salt and pepper.

Ping your grains in the microwave according to packet instructions.

Come back to the carrots. Stir in the almonds and the mixed grains, spoon onto a plate and drizzle over the coriander dressing.

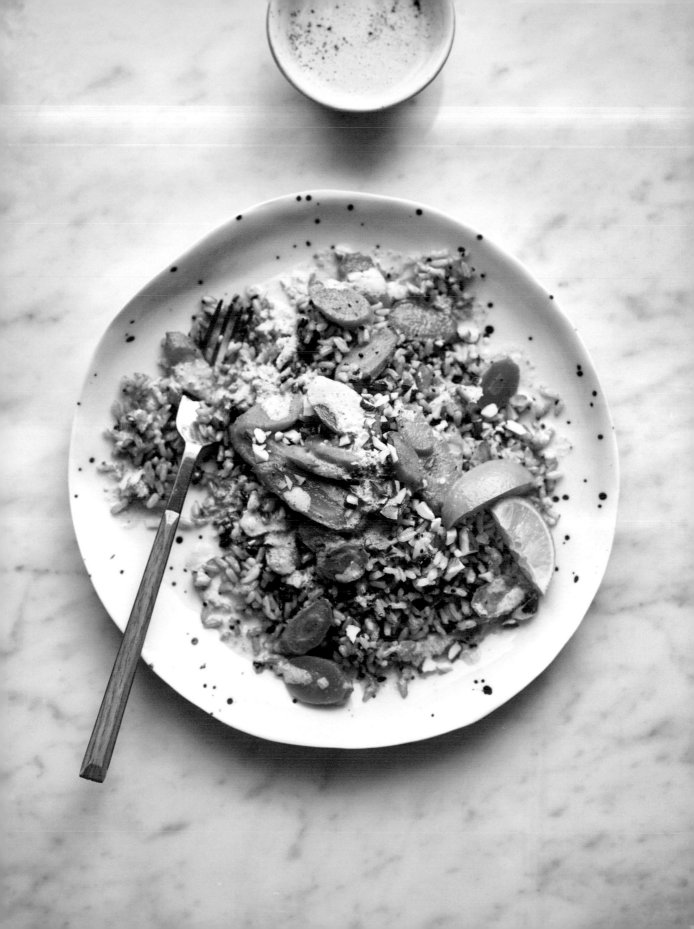

SERVES 1

MAKE AHEAD

Ingredients

100g frozen peas
1 small avocado, de-stoned
handful of mint
2 pre-cooked beetroots
150g pre-cooked puy lentils
1 tbsp sherry vinegar
salt and pepper
handful of pea shoots
50g feta
1 tbsp toasted flaked almonds
drizzle of olive oil

Beetroot, avocado and pea lentil bowl

Method

Put the frozen peas in a microwaveable bowl along with 1 tablespoon of water. Cover with cling film, then zap on high for a minute to defrost.

Slice the avocado, pick the mint leaves, then cut your beetroot into wedges.

Ping your lentils in the microwave according to packet instructions, then tip into a bowl and stir through the vinegar along with a generous pinch of salt and pepper.

Place the avocado, peas, beetroot and pea shoots on top of the lentils. Crumble over the feta, scatter with flaked almonds and mint, then drizzle with olive oil to serve.

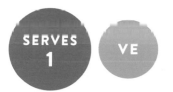

SERVES 1 · VE

Pecan, apple and kale quinoa salad with tahini dressing

MAKE AHEAD

Ingredients

60g uncooked quinoa
2 large handfuls of kale,
  stalks removed
juice of 1 lemon
big pinch of dried chilli flakes
salt and pepper
1 apple, cored
2 tbsp tahini
30g toasted pecans, roughly
  chopped
handful of dill, chopped

Method

Bring a kettle of water to the boil.

Put the quinoa into a medium saucepan, pour over plenty of boiling water and cook for 15 minutes, or according to packet instructions.

Meanwhile, place the kale in a medium serving bowl and squeeze half the lemon juice over the top. Sprinkle over the chilli flakes along with some salt and pepper, then massage it all together – this will soften the kale.

Slice the apple, then squeeze over a little lemon juice to stop it from going brown.

Make the creamy dressing by whisking the remaining lemon juice into the tahini with 2 tablespoons of water and a good pinch of salt and pepper.

Drain the quinoa, then tip into the bowl with the kale. Stir through the tahini dressing so that all the grains get coated, then mix in the apple, pecans and dill.

SERVES 1

Vietnamese noodle salad

MAKE AHEAD
Add the egg just before serving.

Ingredients

120g dried rice noodles
1 egg
juice of 1 lime
1 tbsp soy sauce
1 tsp soft brown sugar
1 tsp rice wine vinegar
½ red chilli, finely chopped –
   remove the seeds if you don't
   like it hot
1 small clove garlic, finely
   chopped
1 carrot, peeled and grated
1 courgette, grated
2 tbsp salted roasted peanuts,
   roughly chopped
handful of mint leaves

Method

Bring a kettle of water to the boil.

Put the rice noodles into a bowl. Pour over enough boiling water to cover, then stir and leave for about 3 minutes until softened.

Pour the remaining water into a saucepan and bring to the boil. Lower the heat on the saucepan, so the water is hissing rather than bubbling, then lower in your egg. Cook for 6 minutes.

While your egg is cooking, mix the lime juice, soy sauce, soft brown sugar, rice wine vinegar, chilli and garlic together for your dressing.

Come back to your noodles. Drain them into a colander then rinse under cold water until completely cool. Separate the noodles with your fingers. Shake off any excess water, then tip them into your serving bowl and stir through the dressing, grated carrot and courgette.

By now your egg should be cooked. Remove with a slotted spoon and rinse under cold water until cool enough to handle. Peel, then cut in half.

Top the noodles with the soft-boiled egg, then scatter over the roasted peanuts and mint.

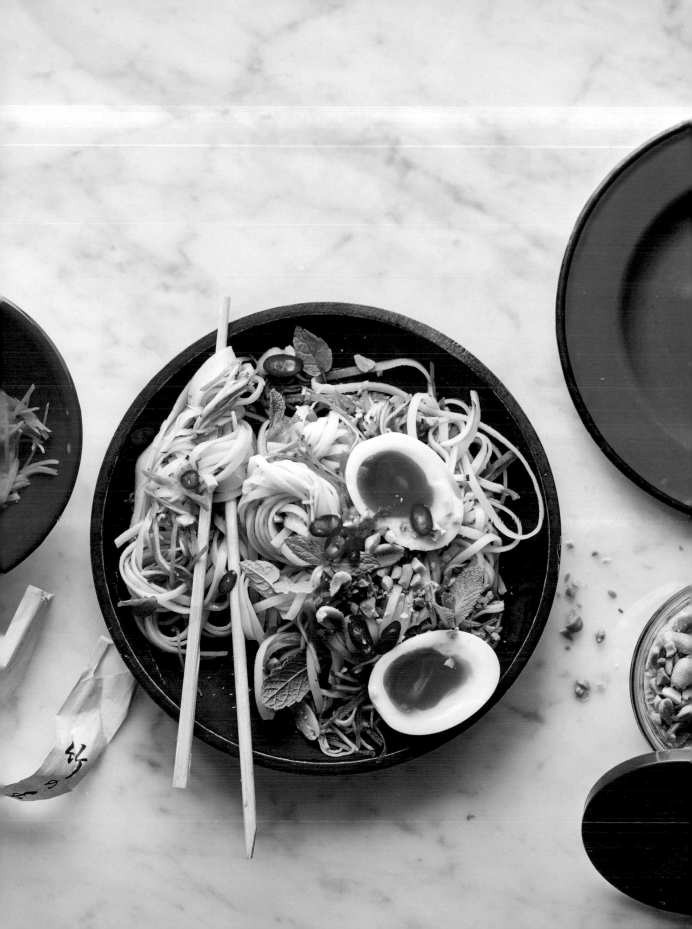

MAKE AHEAD

Ingredients

½ head of cauliflower (you can use leftovers from the cauliflower steak on page 85)

2 tbsp olive oil

1 tsp ground cumin

1 tsp mustard seeds

big pinch of dried chilli flakes

salt and pepper

100g frozen peas

100g frozen broad beans

30g hazelnuts

handful of parsley, chopped

handful of mint leaves, chopped

juice of ½ lemon

Warm cauliflower tabbouleh

Method

Preheat the oven to 220°C (fan 200°C/gas mark 7). Put a small saucepan of water on to boil.

Roughly chop the cauliflower, then blitz in a food processor until it resembles couscous. Tip into a bowl, then stir through 1 tablespoon of the olive oil with the ground cumin, mustard seeds, chilli flakes and a generous pinch of salt.

Spread the cauliflower 'couscous' out into an even layer on a baking tray. Roast for 10 minutes, stirring halfway.

While the 'couscous' is cooking, drop the peas and broad beans into the boiling water. Cook for 2 minutes, then drain into a sieve.

Toast the hazelnuts in a dry frying pan over a medium heat until smelling nutty, then allow to cool and roughly chop.

Take the cauliflower out of the oven. Tip it into your bowl, stir through the cooked peas and broad beans, toasted hazelnuts, parsley, mint and remaining olive oil. Squeeze in the lemon juice and season with salt and pepper to taste.

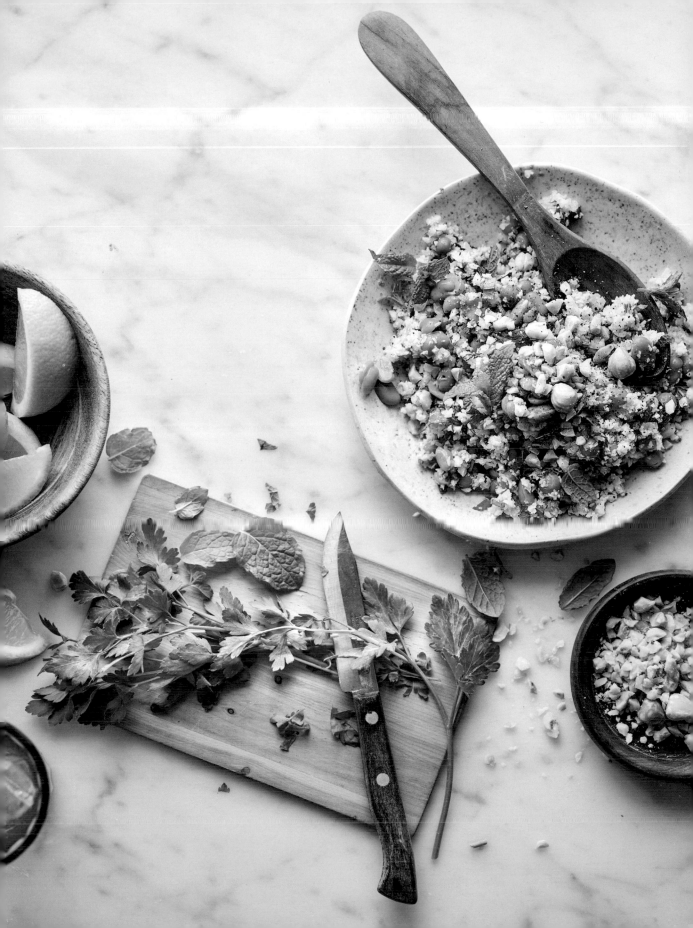

Spicy fried rice and mango salad

MAKE AHEAD

Ingredients

½ red chilli, de-seeded and
 finely chopped
100g fresh mango, cut into cubes
handful of coriander, chopped,
 plus a few sprigs to serve
juice of ½ lime
salt and pepper
1 tbsp coconut oil
2 spring onions, finely sliced
1–1½ tbsp jerk paste or jerk
 seasoning – depending on
 how spicy you like it
150g pre-cooked wholegrain rice
200g kidney beans, drained
 and rinsed
dollop of coconut yoghurt,
 to serve

Method

Mix the chilli and mango in a bowl with the coriander, lime juice and salt and pepper to taste. Mango salsa – done.

Next, melt the coconut oil in a frying pan over a medium heat. Chuck in the sliced spring onions and cook for 1 minute or so until softened. Spoon in the jerk paste and cook, stirring for 1 minute until smelling fragrant.

Add the rice and use the back of your spoon to break up any grains of rice that are stuck together. Give it a good stir, then mix in the kidney beans and a few splashes of water to loosen everything. Fry until heated through.

Scrape the spicy fried rice into your bowl. Top with the mango salsa, a few coriander sprigs and a dollop of coconut yoghurt.

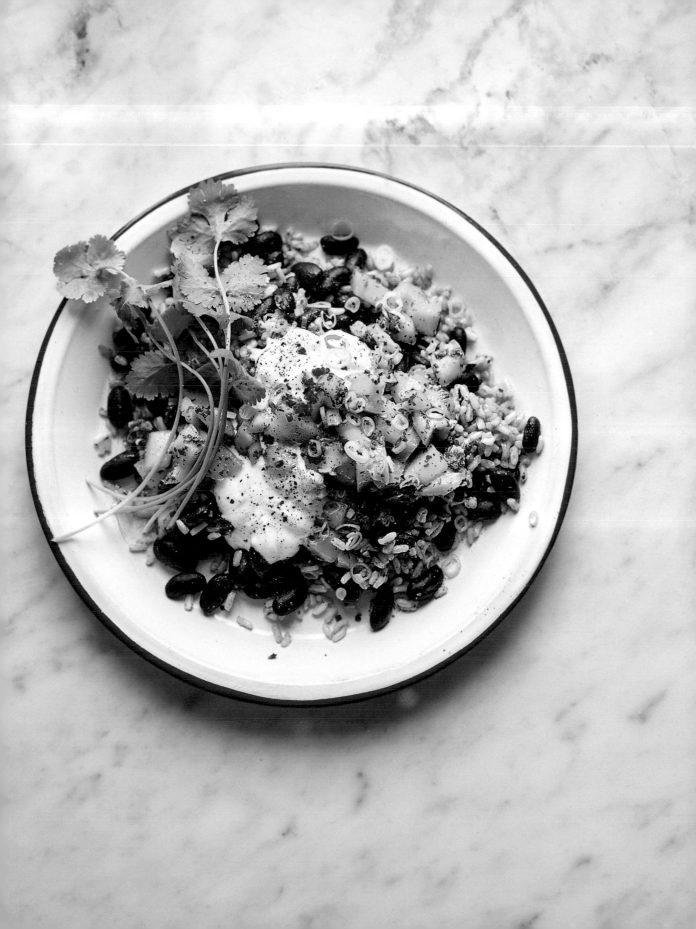

Breaded goat's cheese with pesto, sugarsnaps and watercress

Ingredients

30g walnuts, roughly chopped
½ small bunch basil,
  leaves only
3 tbsp olive oil
1 tbsp sherry vinegar
salt and pepper
1 egg
50g breadcrumbs
50g firm goat's cheese, cut into
  four rounds
big handful of watercress
100g sugarsnap peas
5 cherry tomatoes, halved –
  I like a mix of yellow and red

Method

Toast the walnuts in a dry frying pan for a few minutes, then allow to cool and roughly chop. Set aside the frying pan to use later.

Tip half the walnuts into a small food processor with the basil leaves, 2 tablespoons of the olive oil and the sherry vinegar. Pour in a splash of water and a good pinch of salt and pepper, then blitz to smooth pesto. Add a little more water if you need it.

Crack the egg into a shallow bowl and whisk with a fork. Tip the breadcrumbs into a separate bowl. Dunk the goat's cheese slices first into the egg, then coat them in the breadcrumbs.

Heat the remaining olive oil in your frying pan over a medium to high heat. Add the goat's cheese and fry for 2 minutes on each side until golden and oozy.

Pile the watercress, sugarsnap peas and tomatoes onto your plate. Stir in the pesto, then top with the hot cheese. Scatter over the remaining walnuts and get stuck in.

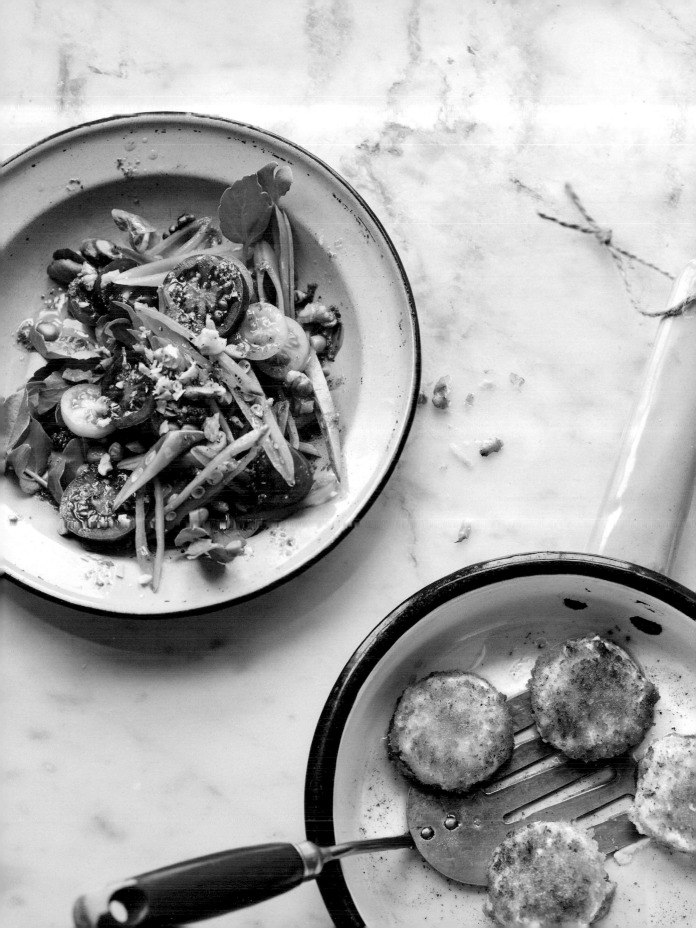

Tex Mex corn and sweet potato salad

SERVES 1

Ingredients

1 sweet potato, skin on, cut
   into small pieces
½ lime, cut into wedges
1 tbsp coconut oil
1 tsp ground cumin
1 tsp chilli powder
1 x 200g tin of sweetcorn,
   drained
120g halloumi, sliced
2 tomatoes, chopped
   into chunks
handful of coriander,
   roughly chopped
salt and pepper
½ avocado, de-stoned and sliced
15g bag of salted popcorn
   – optional

Method

Put the sweet potato and lime wedges in a microwaveable bowl. Cover with cling film, then zap on high for 10 minutes until completely cooked.

While the sweet potato is cooking, melt the coconut oil in a frying pan over a high heat. Sprinkle in the cumin and chilli powder and cook for 30 seconds until fragrant, then tip in the sweetcorn. Fry for 2 minutes to cook off the water left in the sweetcorn, then tip into a bowl.

Put the frying pan back on a high heat (don't bother washing it – extra flavour). Lay in the halloumi slices and fry for 2 minutes on each side until the cheese is super crisp.

Meanwhile, mix the tomatoes and coriander through the sweetcorn mix. Come back to the sweet potato, which should now be cooked. Remove the lime, squeeze the juice out over the sweet potato, then stir through the sweetcorn salad. Season everything with salt and pepper then pile onto a plate.

Lay the avocado and halloumi slices on top of the salad then scatter over the popcorn, for extra crunch, if using.

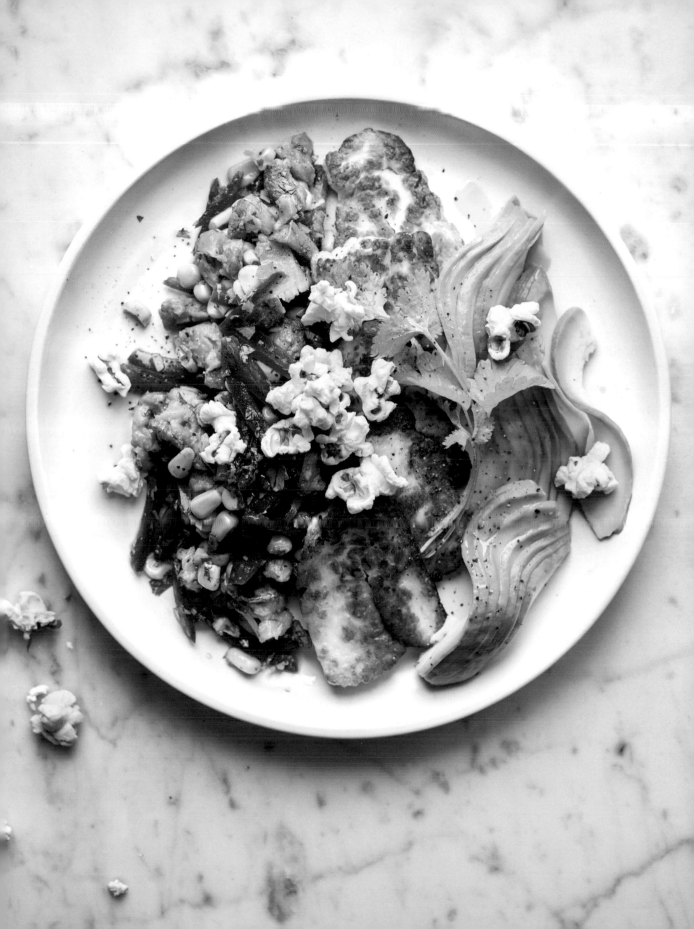

MAKE AHEAD
Keep the pitta separate so it
stays crisp.

Ingredients

1 pitta bread
2 tbsp olive oil
2 tsp za'atar
salt
8 cherry tomatoes – I like
  a mix of yellow and red
handful of mint
handful of parsley
5 radishes
½ cucumber
1 spring onion
2 tbsp pomegranate seeds
50g feta, crumbled
juice of ½ lemon

Tomato and pomegranate fattoush

Method

Preheat the oven to 200°C (fan 180°C/gas mark 6).

Using scissors, cut the pitta into random shards. Transfer to a flat baking sheet, then toss with ½ tablespoon olive oil, 1 teaspoon of the za'atar and a good pinch of salt. Spread out in a single layer and roast in the oven for 10 minutes, turning halfway, until golden and crisp.

While the pitta is roasting, chop the rest of your ingredients. Halve the cherry tomatoes, pick the mint leaves and roughly chop along with the parsley. Cut the radishes into quarters. Halve the cucumber lengthways, then use a teaspoon to remove the seeds and chop. Finely slice the spring onion. Put all these ingredients into a serving bowl along with the pomegranate seeds and the crumbled feta.

For the dressing, whisk together the lemon juice, remaining olive oil and za'atar and a good pinch of salt. Pour this over the other ingredients and mix well to combine.

Get your pitta out of the oven and mix it through the salad. Fattoush done.

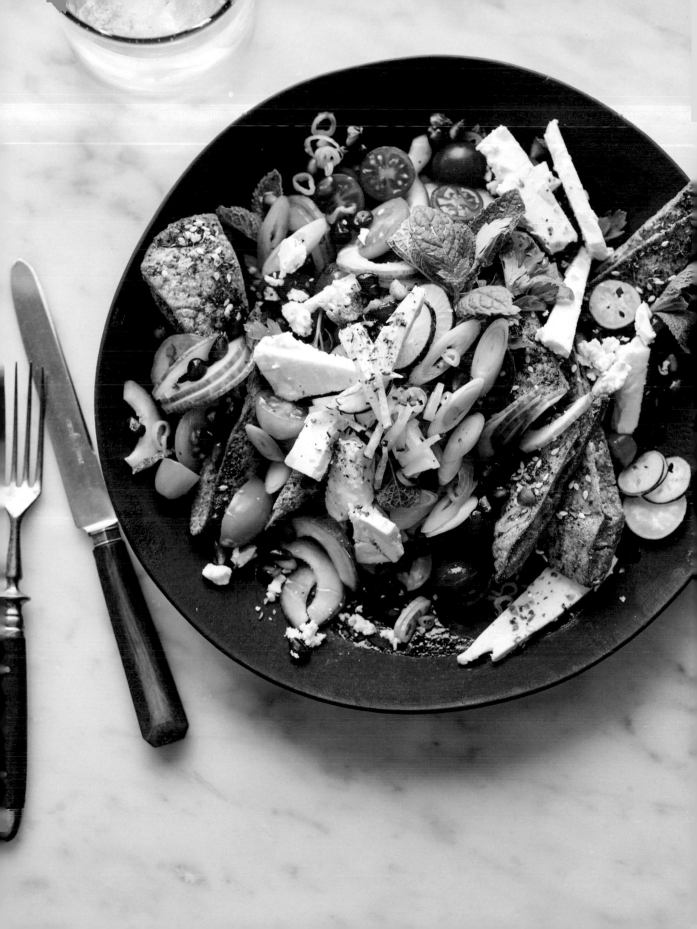

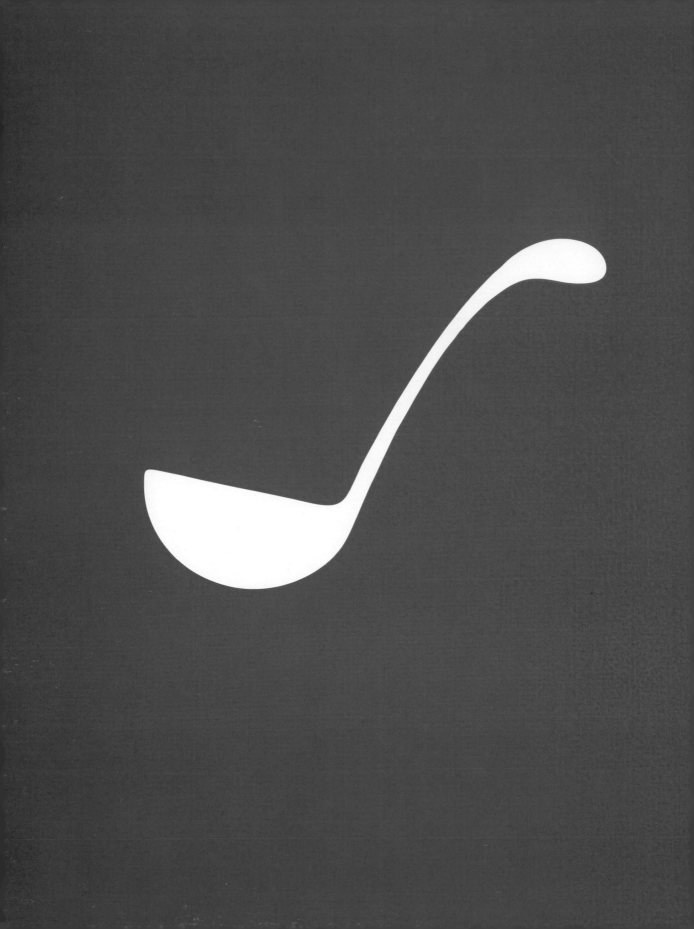

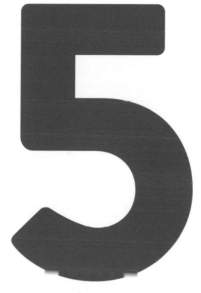

SOUPS
AND STEWS

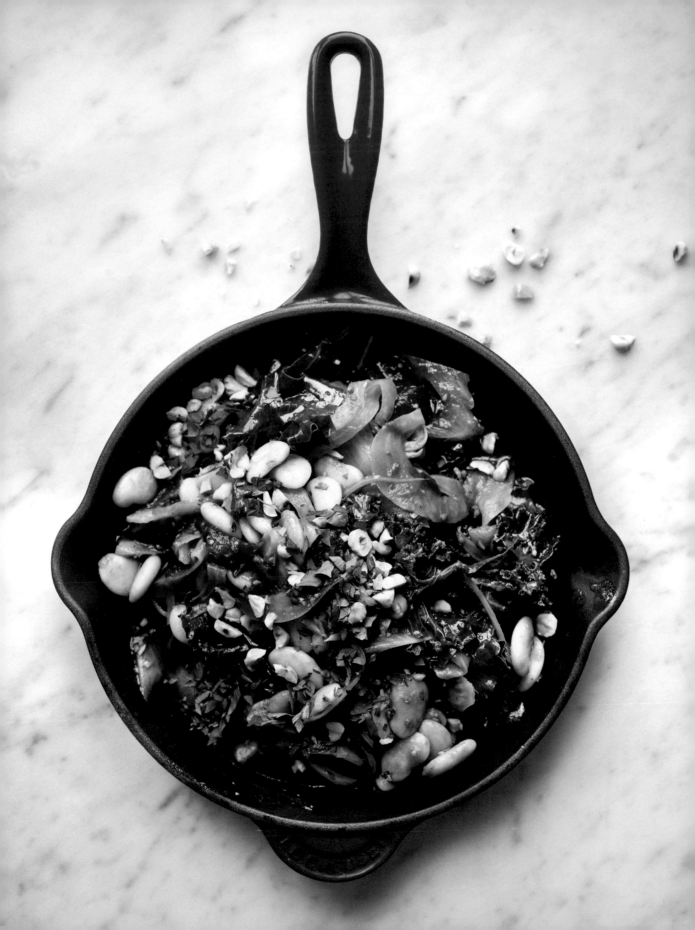

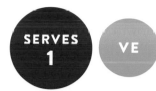

SERVES 1

VE

Ingredients

1 tbsp coconut oil
1 fennel bulb, finely sliced
salt and pepper
2 cloves garlic
½ red chilli
handful of parsley
 (stalks and all)
zest and juice of ½ lemon
1 x 400g tin of cherry tomatoes
1 x 400g tin of butterbeans,
 drained and rinsed
1 tbsp hazelnuts
big handful of kale, stalks
 removed

Kale, fennel and butterbean stew

Method

Melt the coconut oil in a saucepan over a medium to high heat. Add the fennel and a pinch of salt. Cook for 4 minutes, until softened.

Meanwhile, finely chop the garlic, chilli and parsley stalks. Once the fennel has softened, add these to the pan along with the lemon zest. Cook for 1 minute until it smells fragrant.

Tip in the cherry tomatoes and butterbeans along with some salt and pepper. Give everything a good stir. Bring the stew to a boil, then simmer away for 5 minutes.

While the stew is cooking, toast the hazelnuts in a dry small frying pan, then allow to cool and roughly chop with the parsley leaves.

Stir the kale into the stew. When it has wilted, squeeze in the lemon juice and spoon the stew into a bowl. Scatter over the chopped hazelnuts and parsley leaves.

Smokey tomato and pepper stew with pesto butterbean mash

MAKE AHEAD
GOOD TO FREEZE

Ingredients

1 tbsp olive oil

1 red onion, finely sliced

salt and pepper

1 tsp smoked paprika

1 x 400g tin of cherry tomatoes

200g butterbeans, drained
and rinsed

2 tbsp basil pesto (fresh is best
for this recipe)

1 jarred roasted red pepper,
drained and sliced

splash of sherry or red
wine vinegar

Method

Pour the olive oil into a saucepan over a medium heat. Add the onion and a pinch of salt, then cook for 5 minutes until softened. Sprinkle in the smoked paprika, cook for 1 minute more, then tip in the tin of cherry tomatoes. Leave to bubble away.

In a separate small saucepan, add the butterbeans, basil pesto and 50ml water. Place over a low heat (you are just warming the beans through). Roughly mash the warmed beans with a potato masher or a fork.

Come back to the stew. Stir in the roasted red pepper and season with salt, pepper and vinegar to taste.

Pile the pesto mash into a bowl, ladle the tomato pepper stew alongside and tuck into this bowl of comfort food.

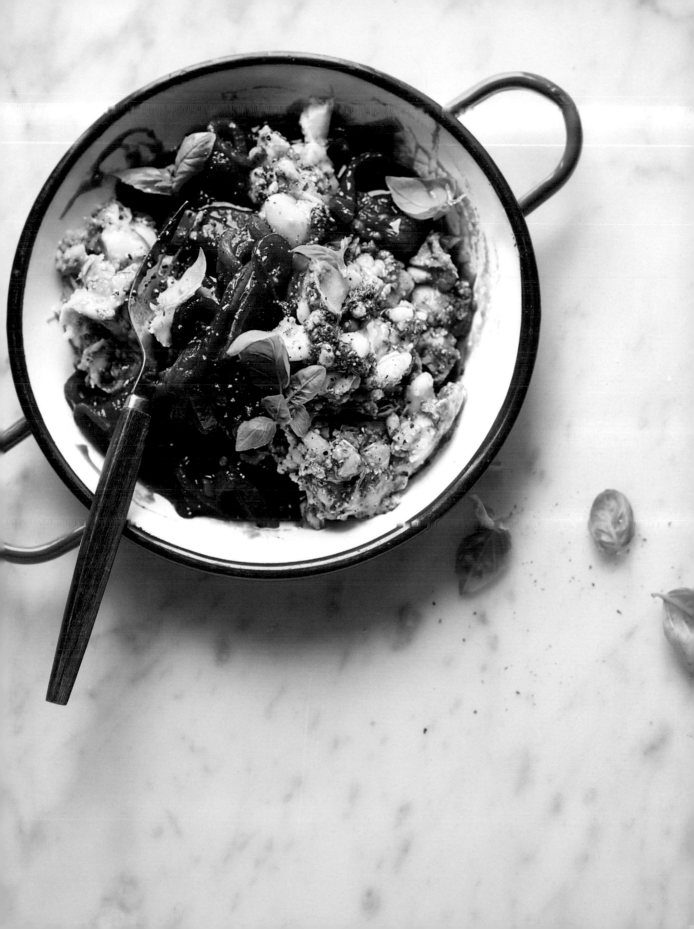

**MAKE AHEAD
GOOD TO FREEZE**

Ingredients

1 tbsp olive oil

1 fat clove garlic, crushed

big pinch of dried chilli flakes

½ bunch of basil, leaves
 picked and stalks
 finely sliced

200g chopped tinned tomatoes
 (½ tin)

100g tinned cannellini beans,
 drained and rinsed

salt and pepper

1 slice sourdough bread –
 the staler the better

splash of red wine vinegar

1 tbsp sundried tomato pesto

1 tbsp ricotta

Tuscan bread soup

Method

Put the olive oil in a saucepan over a medium heat. Add the garlic, chilli flakes and basil stalks. Cook for 30 seconds or so until the garlic has turned golden.

Tip in the chopped tomatoes, cannellini beans and most of the basil leaves along with a good pinch of salt and pepper. Bring the soup to a boil. Tear in the bread – if it isn't very stale, toast it briefly first. Cook on high for 10 minutes.

Take the pan off the heat, stir in the red wine vinegar and 100ml cold water, then blitz with a soup blender or in a food processor, adding a splash of water if the soup is too thick.

Spoon into a bowl, swirl through the pesto and top with the ricotta and remaining basil leaves.

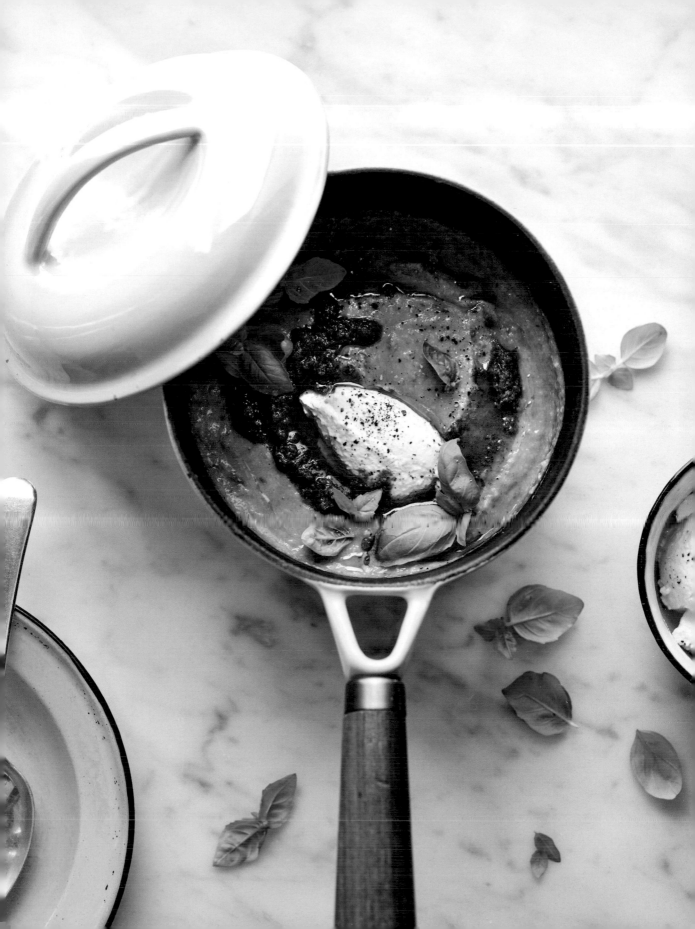

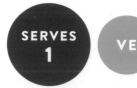

SERVES 1 **VE**

MAKE AHEAD
GOOD TO FREEZE

Ingredients

1 tbsp coconut oil
½ onion, finely chopped
salt and pepper
2 tsp garlic–ginger paste
½ tsp ground turmeric
1 tsp garam masala
2 tomatoes, roughly chopped
1 x 400g tin of chickpeas
2 handfuls of spinach leaves
squeeze of lemon juice
handful of coriander leaves
coconut yoghurt, to serve
 – optional

Chickpea, tomato and spinach curry

Method

Melt the coconut oil in a saucepan over a low heat. Chuck in the onion, along with a pinch of salt. Cook for 6 minutes until soft.

Stir in the garlic–ginger paste, turmeric and garam masala. Cook for 1 minute, stirring until it smells fragrant.

Turn up the heat, chuck in the tomatoes and the tin of chickpeas with all of their water. Season with a good pinch of salt and pepper, then leave the curry to bubble away for 5 minutes.

Drop in the spinach leaves. Once wilted, take the pan off the heat and squeeze in the lemon juice to taste. Spoon into a bowl, stir through most of the coriander leaves, then top with the rest. Serve with coconut yoghurt, if you like.

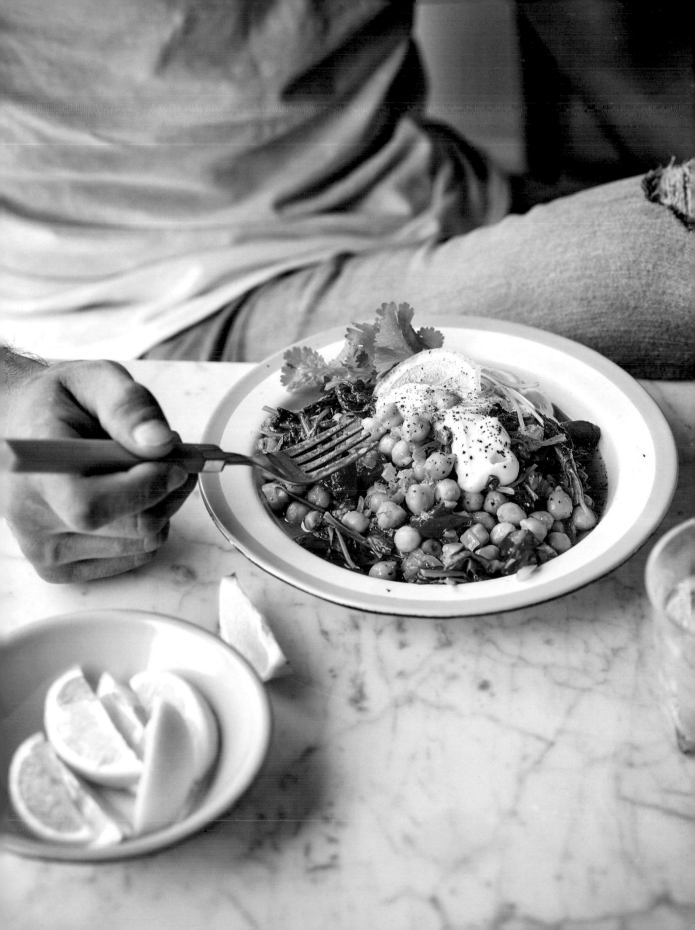

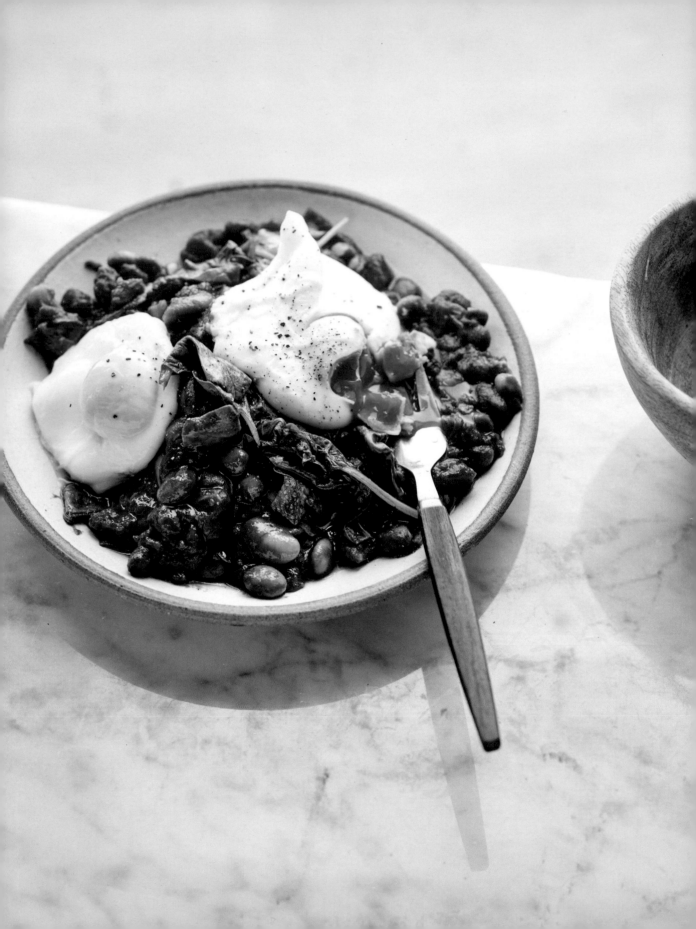

SERVES 1

Moroccan bean stew with poached eggs

Ingredients

- 1 x 400g tin of chopped tomatoes
- 1 x 400g tin of mixed beans, drained and rinsed
- ¼ tsp ground cinnamon
- ½–1 tsp smoked paprika
- 1 tsp ground cumin
- salt and pepper
- 2 eggs
- 2 large handfuls of spinach leaves

Method

Bring a saucepan of water to the boil.

Tip the tin of chopped tomatoes into a saucepan along with the beans, cinnamon, paprika and cumin together with some salt and pepper. Bring to the boil, then simmer the stew away for 10 minutes, stirring regularly until it has thickened.

Come back to your saucepan of boiling water. Turn down the heat until the water is just burping. Crack the eggs straight into the water. Poach for 3–4 minutes or until the white has set but the yolk is still runny, then carefully lift out with a slotted spoon and drain on kitchen roll.

Stir the spinach through the bean stew. When wilted, spoon into a bowl and top with the poached eggs and a good pinch of salt and pepper.

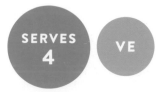

LONGER RECIPE
MAKE AHEAD
Keep for up to 3 days in the fridge.
GOOD TO FREEZE
Only the dal, not the cauliflower
cashew topping.

Ingredients

3 tbsp coconut oil
1 heaped tbsp garlic–ginger
   paste
1 green chilli, finely chopped
350g red split lentils
1½ tsp ground turmeric
1 head of cauliflower,
   florets only
1 tsp garam masala
2 tsp mustard seeds
2 tsp cumin seeds
salt
120g cashew nuts
large handful of cherry
   tomatoes, halved – I like
   a mix of yellow and red
200g baby spinach leaves
squeeze of lemon juice

Cauliflower, cashew nut and spinach dal

Method

Melt 1 tablespoon of the coconut oil in a large saucepan.
Stir in the garlic–ginger paste and green chilli. Cook for
1 minute until it smells fragrant, then tip in the lentils and
ground turmeric. Give everything a good stir so that the
lentils get nicely coated in the yellow spice mix.

Pour enough cold water into the pan to completely cover the
lentils. The water needs to reach around 5cm above the surface
of the lentils. Bring to the boil then turn down the heat so
that the water is just burping. Simmer for 30 minutes, stirring
occasionally, until the lentils are completely softened and
have absorbed a lot of the water. If it looks dry at any point
top up with more water.

While the dal is simmering, preheat the oven to 220°C
(fan 200°C, gas mark 7). Cut the cauliflower into smallish
florets. Melt the remaining coconut oil in a large bowl in the
microwave, then stir in the garam masala, mustard seeds and
cumin seeds along with some salt. Drop in the cauliflower
and toss so that each floret gets coated in the spices.

Tip the cauliflower onto a large baking tray and roast in the
oven. After 15 minutes, tip the cashews into the baking tray.
Return to the oven for 10 minutes so that the nuts toast along
with the cauliflower.

Come back to your dal, which should now be cooked and the
consistency of wet porridge. Stir in the cherry tomatoes and
spinach. When the spinach has wilted, squeeze in the lemon
juice and season with salt to taste.

Spoon the dal into bowls and top with the spiced cauliflower
and cashew nuts, making sure you scrape all the tasty bits
from the tray into your bowls.

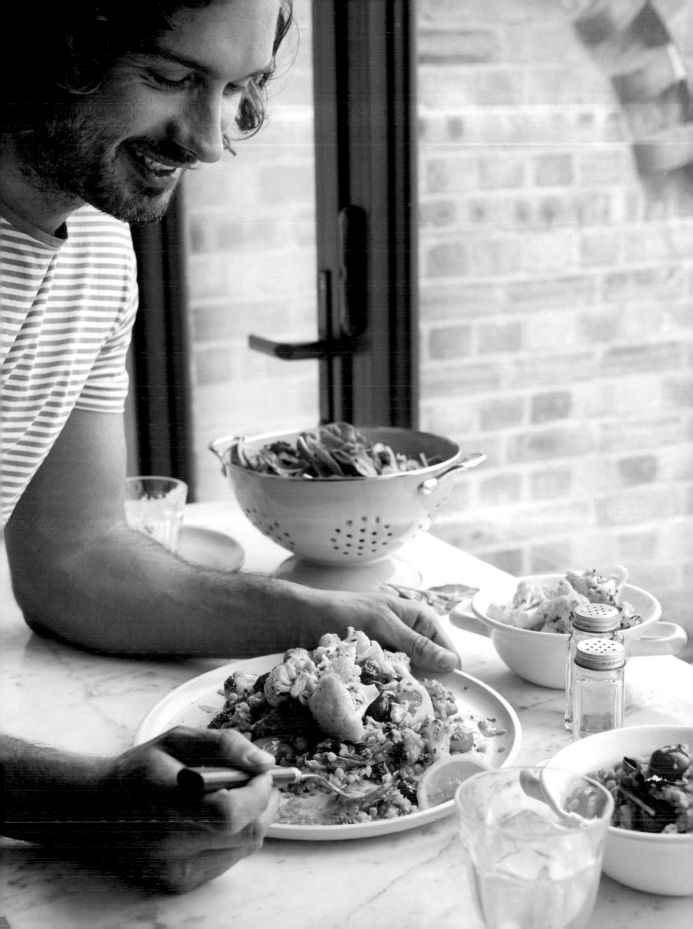

**SERVES
2**

Hearty veg and potato stew

LONGER RECIPE

Ingredients

2 big potatoes, peeled and
cut into quarters

4 tbsp butter

2 fat leeks, trimmed and finely
sliced into half-moons

salt and pepper

2 cloves garlic, finely chopped

200g frozen peas

2 big handfuls of kale, stalks
removed

100ml white wine

100ml double cream

1 tbsp wholegrain mustard

60g mature cheddar, grated

Method

Bring a kettle of water to the boil, then pour into a medium
saucepan. Drop the potato chunks into the water and cook
for 20 minutes until the potato is completely soft.

Meanwhile, melt 2 tablespoons of the butter in a large
ovenproof frying pan over a medium heat. Chuck in your
leeks along with a pinch of salt and cook for 10 minutes
until they have collapsed and are soft.

Add the garlic, cook for 1 minute more, then drop in the
peas and kale and cook, stirring, until the kale has just
wilted. Turn down the heat to low and season to taste.

Whisk the white wine, double cream, 50ml water and
mustard together in a jug. Pour this into the pan with
your leeks.

Preheat your grill to maximum. Drain your potatoes and
transfer them back into their pan. Add the remaining
butter and mash. Stir through half the grated cheese and
season to taste.

Spoon the mash on top of your creamy veg, then use the
back of your spoon to spread it out into a thin layer across
the top of the pan – don't worry if some of the veg pokes
through around the edge. Sprinkle the rest of the cheese on
top. Whack under the grill for 5–10 minutes until golden
brown, oozing and cheesy. Take out of the grill and leave to
rest for 5 minutes, then spoon into two bowls.

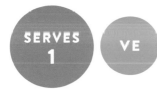

SERVES 1 · **VE**

MAKE AHEAD
Add the tofu when you reheat.

Ingredients

1 miso soup sachet

5g dried mushrooms, such as shitake

1 tbsp coconut oil

1 tsp garlic–ginger paste

2 spring onions, finely sliced (green bits and all)

100g chestnut mushrooms, cut into quarters

1 pak choi, cut into quarters

1 tbsp soy sauce

100g silken tofu, chopped into 2cm cubes

1 tsp sesame seeds

Miso mushroom soup

Method

Bring a kettle of water to the boil. Tip the contents of the miso soup sachet and the dried mushrooms into a jug. When the kettle has boiled, pour in 400ml boiling water, then leave the mushrooms to rehydrate.

Meanwhile, melt the coconut oil in a saucepan. Stir in the garlic–ginger paste. Cook for 1 minute until it smells fragrant, then stir in three-quarters of the spring onions and chestnut mushrooms. Fry for 5 minutes until all the liquid has come out of the mushrooms.

Pour the miso–mushroom stock into the saucepan. Bring back to the boil, then drop in the pak choi. Cook for 2 minutes until tender, then stir in the soy sauce.

Spoon the soup into a bowl. Top with the silken tofu and remaining spring onion. Scatter over the sesame seeds.

SERVES 1

Ingredients

1 sweet potato, peeled and
  cut into chunks
1½ tbsp olive oil
salt and pepper
½ red onion, finely sliced
1 red pepper, sliced
1 clove garlic, crushed
2 tsp chipotle paste
½ tsp ground cumin
1 x 400g tin of chopped
  tomatoes
400g kidney beans, drained
  and rinsed
dollop of sour cream
a few coriander leaves and
  grated cheddar, to serve

Smokey sweet potato chilli

Method

Preheat the oven to 220°C (fan 200°C, gas mark 7).

Put your sweet potato on a baking tray. Mix with ½ tablespoon of the olive oil and some salt and pepper. Spread out into a single layer so it cooks evenly, then whack in the oven for 20 minutes.

While your sweet potato is cooking, pour the remaining oil into a saucepan over a medium heat. Tip in the sliced red onion and red pepper, along with a pinch of salt and cook for 7 minutes until soft. Add the garlic, chipotle paste and ground cumin to the pan.

Give everything a good stir, then cook for 1 minute until it smells fragrant.

Pour in the chopped tomatoes and kidney beans. Simmer away for 10 minutes.

Come back to your sweet potato, which should now be soft. Scrape it into the chilli, then season to taste.

Spoon the chilli into your bowl, dollop on the sour cream, then top with a few coriander leaves and the grated cheese.

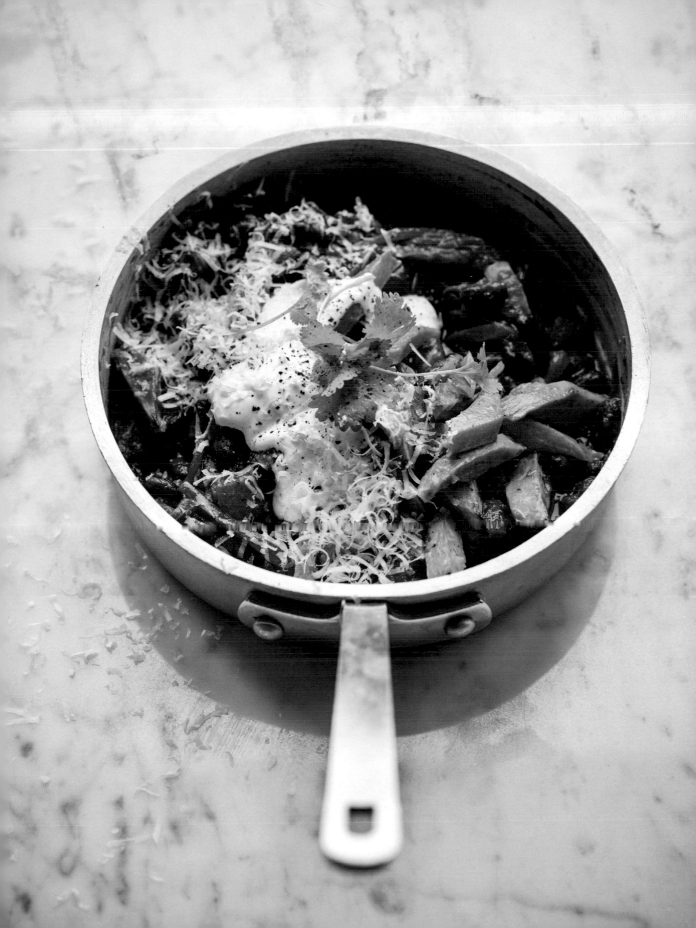

SERVES 1

Creamy beetroot mustardy lentils

Ingredients

1 tbsp coconut oil
½ onion, finely chopped
salt
30g walnuts
1 clove garlic, finely chopped
200g pre-cooked puy lentils
1–2 tsp dijon mustard
50ml double cream
handful of parsley,
  roughly chopped, plus a
  little extra to serve
2 ready-cooked beetroot,
  cut into wedges
squeeze of lemon juice

Method

Melt the coconut oil in a saucepan over a medium heat. Add the onion along with a pinch of salt. Cook for 8 minutes until soft.

While the onion is cooking, toast the walnuts in a dry small frying pan over a medium heat, then allow to cool and roughly chop.

Stir the garlic into the onion pan. Cook for a minute, until it smells fragrant. Tip in the lentils, breaking them up with the back of your spoon. Give everything a good stir, then mix in the dijon mustard, double cream and 2 tablespoons of water. When it is bubbling hot, remove from the heat and mix in the parsley and beetroot. Squeeze in the lemon juice to taste.

Pile the creamy lentils into a bowl. Scatter over the toasted walnuts and remaining parsley.

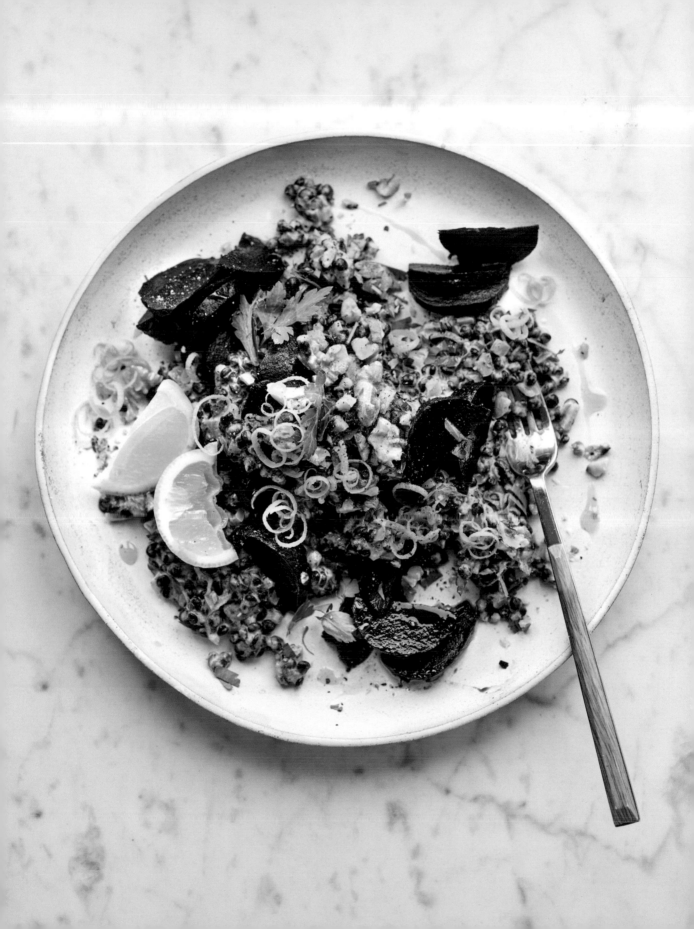

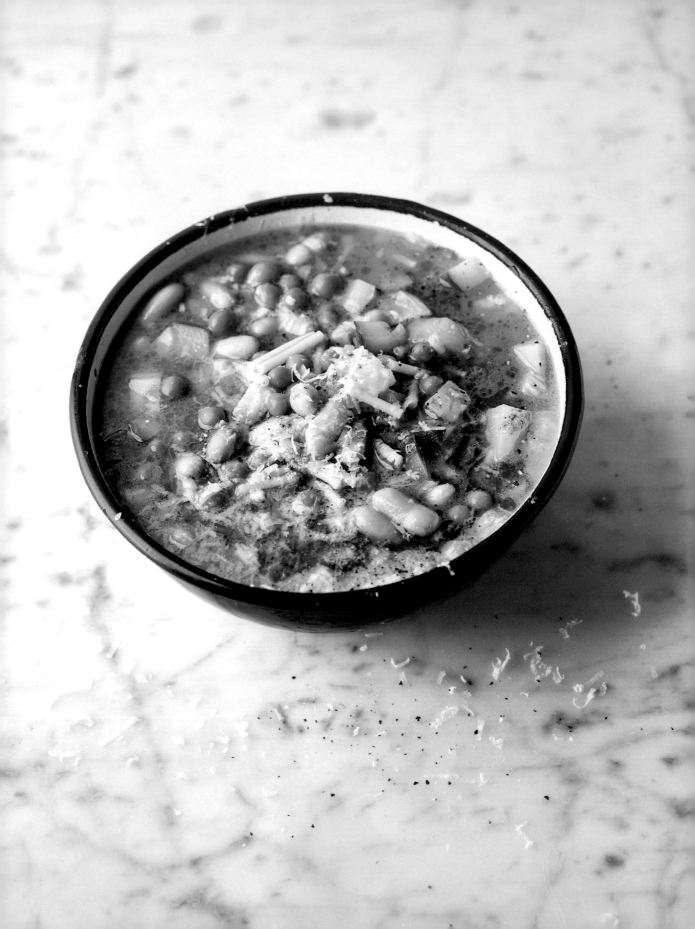

SERVES 1

Courgette, pea and pesto minestrone

MAKE AHEAD

Ingredients

1 tbsp olive oil
½ onion, finely chopped
1 courgette, finely chopped
1 fat clove garlic, finely
  chopped
salt
400ml hot veg stock
60g spaghetti
200g haricot or cannellini
  beans, drained and rinsed
50g frozen peas
2 tbsp basil pesto (fresh is best)
zest and juice of ½ lemon
30g vegetarian hard cheese,
  grated

Method

Add the olive oil to a saucepan over a medium heat. Add the onion, courgette and garlic along with a pinch of salt. Cook for 5 minutes until mostly softened.

Pour in the stock. Using your hands, break the pasta into small pieces and drop them directly in the pan. Tip in the haricot or cannellini beans. Bring the soup to the boil, then simmer away for 7 minutes until the pasta is pretty much cooked.

Stir in the peas, pesto, lemon zest and juice. Cook for 2 minutes, then spoon the soup into a bowl and top with the grated cheese.

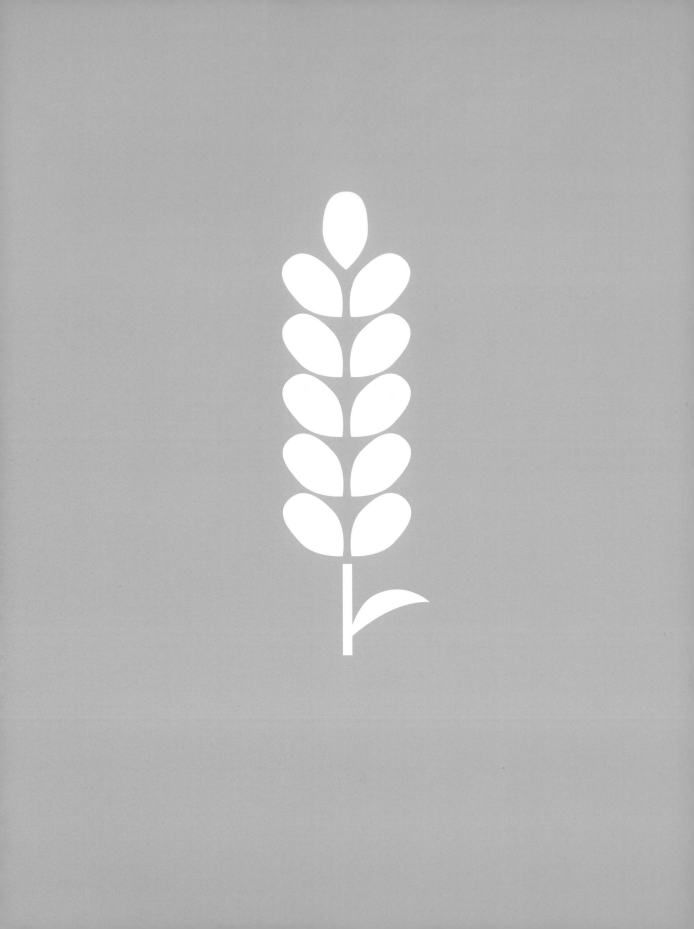

6

PASTA, RICE
AND GRAINS

LONGER RECIPE
MAKE AHEAD
Keep in the fridge for 2–3 days.
GOOD TO FREEZE

Ingredients

2 tbsp olive oil

1 large onion, finely chopped

2 medium carrots, peeled and
   chopped into cubes

salt and pepper

2 cloves garlic, crushed

2 sprigs of rosemary

200g dried green lentils

glass of red wine

2 x 400g tins of chopped
   tomatoes

1 tbsp tomato puree

60g walnuts

1 tbsp balsamic vinegar

cooked pasta of your choice
   and grated cheese, to serve
   – optional

Rosie's beautiful
Bolognese

Method

Add the oil to a saucepan over a low heat. Tip in the
chopped onion and carrots, along with a pinch of salt
and pepper. Cook for 6 minutes until mostly softened.
Stir in the garlic and rosemary sprigs. Cook for another
minute until it smells fragrant, then tip in the lentils.

Give everything a good stir, then pour in the red wine.
When most of the wine has bubbled off, chuck in the
chopped tomatoes, then re-fill one of the tins with water
and pour it in. Stir in the tomato puree then leave to
cook for 20 minutes, until the sauce has thickened
and the lentils are soft.

When the lentils are nearly cooked, toast the walnuts in
a dry frying pan over a medium heat until lightly browned
and smelling nutty. Allow to cool and roughly chop, then
add them to the pan. Stir in the balsamic vinegar and season
your Bolognese to taste, removing the rosemary sprigs.

Serve with cooked pasta and, if you're like me, loads of
grated cheese on top!

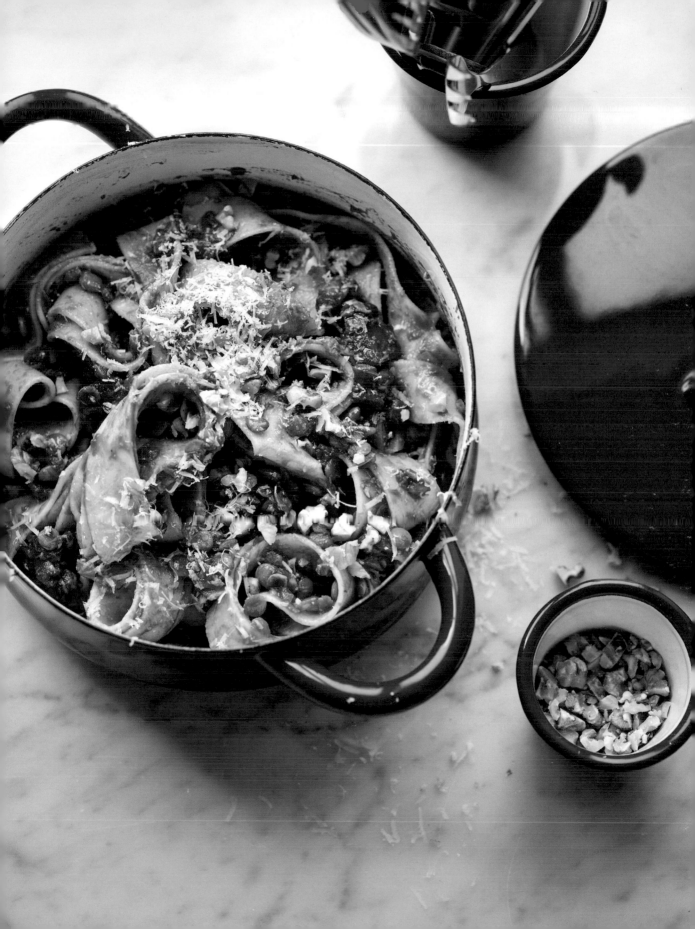

SERVES 1

Lemony pea and yoghurt orzo

MAKE AHEAD

Ingredients

150g frozen peas
100g orzo pasta
75g Greek yoghurt
2 tbsp extra-virgin olive oil
1 small clove garlic
zest and juice of ½ lemon
salt and black pepper
large handful of mint leaves
20g vegetarian hard cheese,
  finely grated – optional

Method

Bring a kettle of water to the boil. Pour a little boiling water over the peas to defrost them and pour the rest into a saucepan ready to cook the orzo.

Drop the orzo into the pan, giving it a good stir so that it doesn't stick together, then cook according to packet instructions.

Drain the peas, then place half in a small food processor with the yoghurt, olive oil, garlic, lemon zest and juice. Season with salt and pepper, then blitz until you have a smooth green pasta sauce.

When the pasta has cooked, drain and return to the pan over a low heat.

Stir through the yoghurt sauce and remaining peas until everything is warmed through, then tip into a bowl, scatter over the mint and top with a good crack of black pepper and some grated cheese, if using.

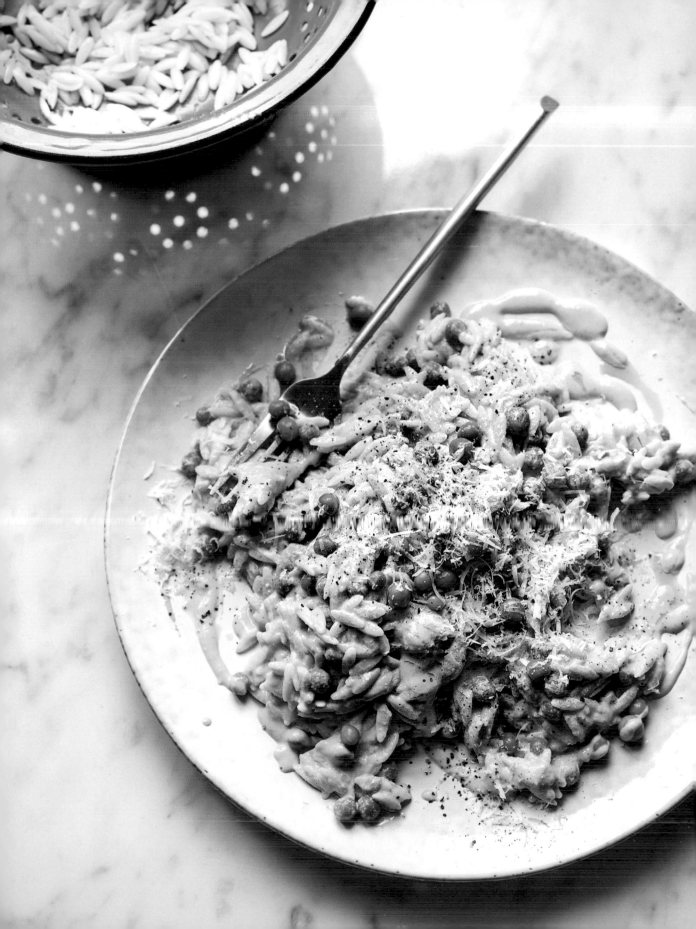

Chargrilled artichoke, lemon, garlic and chilli linguine

Ingredients

- salt and black pepper
- 130g linguine
- 1 pack of chargrilled artichokes, roughly chopped – save the oil from the packet
- 2 cloves garlic, chopped
- 1 red chilli, chopped – remove the seeds if you don't like it hot
- zest and juice of ½ lemon
- 30g pine nuts
- big handful of rocket
- drizzle of olive oil

Method

Bring a large saucepan of water to the boil. Season with salt, then drop in the linguine. Cook for 1 minute less than packet instructions.

While the pasta is cooking, heat the oil from the artichokes in a frying pan over a medium heat. Stir in the garlic and chilli and fry for 1 minute until the garlic is lightly golden – keep watch, you don't want the garlic to burn.

Tip in the artichokes and lemon zest and stir everything well to combine, then push everything to one side of the pan. Scatter the pine nuts onto the clean side. Toast them, then mix with the other ingredients, along with about 50ml of the pasta water. Take the pan off the heat.

Drain the pasta into a colander, then drop into the pan with the artichokes. Squeeze over the lemon juice, then add the rocket and a splash of oil. Toss the whole lot together and season with black pepper. Pile the steaming pasta onto a plate and tuck in.

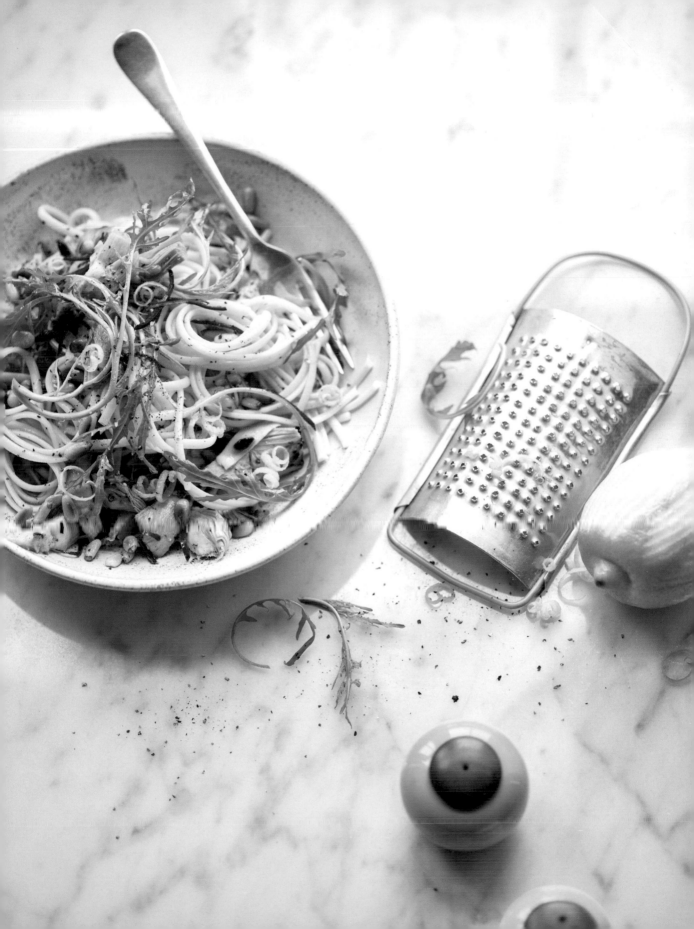

SERVES 1

Baked sundried tomato and mozzarella rice

Ingredients

1 tbsp olive oil
½ red onion, finely sliced
salt
1 courgette, finely chopped
5 sundried tomatoes, chopped
1 clove garlic, finely chopped
big pinch of dried chilli flakes
200g pre-cooked wholegrain
  rice
200ml passata
large handful of baby
  spinach leaves
½ ball of mozzarella (75g)

Method

Preheat the oven to 200°C (fan 180°C, gas mark 6).

Heat the oil in a small ovenproof frying pan over a medium heat. Tip in the onion along with a pinch of salt. Fry for 3 minutes until beginning to soften. Stir in the courgette, sundried tomatoes, garlic and chilli flakes. Fry, stirring regularly, for 5 minutes until the courgette is pretty much cooked.

Add the rice, crumbling it between your fingers as you drop it in along with the passata and about 50ml water. Mix everything together, let the sauce come to the boil, then stir through the spinach.

Take off the heat, break the mozzarella into pieces and dot all over the top of the rice. Bake in the oven for 10 minutes until the cheese is melted and golden.

Carefully remove the pan from the oven (be careful as it will be hot). Let the rice cool for a couple of minutes, then tuck in.

Butternut squash, sage and hazelnut risotto

LONGER RECIPE

Ingredients

½ large butternut squash, cut into small chunks, skin left on

1 tbsp olive oil

1 tsp dried chilli flakes

salt and pepper

1 onion, finely chopped

2 tbsp butter

1 fat clove garlic, finely chopped

180g arborio risotto rice

glass of white wine

800ml veg stock

30g vegetarian hard cheese, finely grated

handful of sage leaves

2 tbsp hazelnuts, roughly chopped

squeeze of lemon juice

Method

Preheat the oven to 220°C (fan 200°C, gas mark 7).

Put the butternut squash on a baking tray and mix with the olive oil, chilli flakes and some salt and pepper. Spread the squash out into a single layer so that it cooks evenly. Roast in the oven for 35 minutes.

While the squash is roasting, put the chopped onion and half the butter in a microwaveable bowl. Cover with cling film, then zap on high for 4 minutes to get soft.

Carefully tip the onion with its butter into a large frying pan over a medium heat. Add the garlic clove and cook for 1 minute until it smells fragrant, then stir in the risotto rice. Give everything a good stir. Glug in the white wine. When the wine has bubbled away, pour in the veg stock.

Simmer the risotto, stirring occasionally so it doesn't stick to the bottom of the pan, until most of the stock has been absorbed by the rice. This usually takes 20 minutes. Keep tasting – you want the rice to be creamy with a little bite, but not crunchy.

Come back to your squash, which should be cooked by now. Scrape it into the risotto along with all the good bits from the bottom of the pan and the grated cheese. Stir, then turn down the heat to its lowest to keep warm. Season to taste.

Now for the fancy bit. Melt the remaining butter in a frying pan. Chuck in the sage leaves and hazelnuts and cook for a minute until the sage leaves start to hiss, then squeeze in the lemon juice. Take off the heat.

Spoon the risotto into two bowls, top with the crispy sage leaves and hazelnuts. Drizzle over the butter and serve.

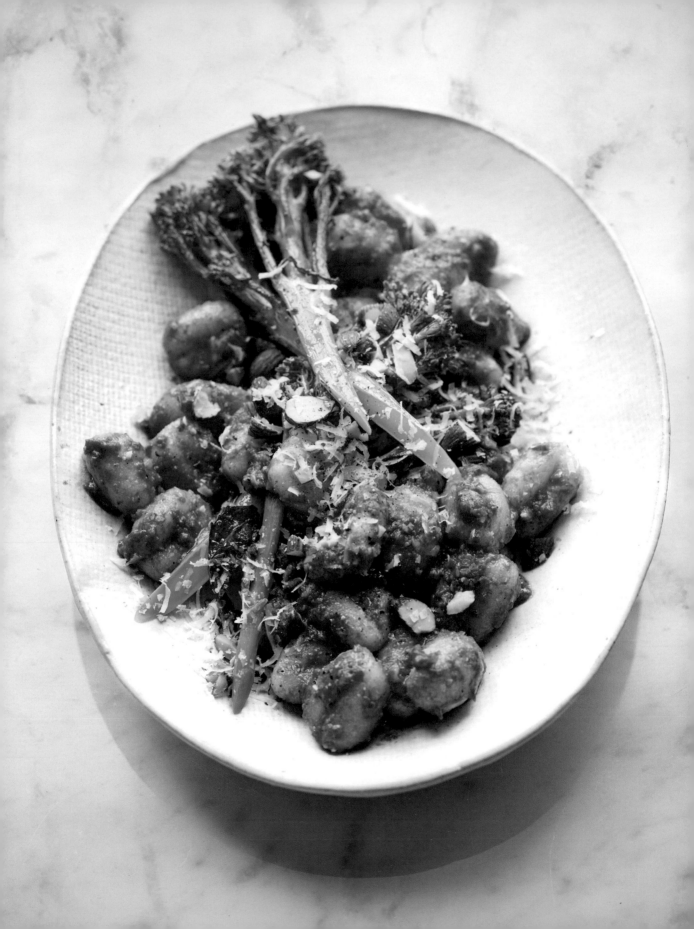

SERVES 1

Gnocchi with midget trees and Romanesco sauce

Ingredients

100g midget trees (tenderstem broccoli), any bigger stalks sliced in half lengthways

2 tbsp olive oil

1 tsp smoked paprika

salt and pepper

50g blanched almonds

1 jarred roasted red pepper, drained and roughly chopped

1 small clove garlic

splash of sherry or red wine vinegar

200g fresh gnocchi

vegetarian hard cheese, to serve – optional

Method

Preheat the oven to 220°C (fan 200°C, gas mark 7) and bring a saucepan of water to the boil.

Put the midget trees on a baking tray and drizzle with a little of the olive oil and a good pinch of smoked paprika. Sprinkle over some salt and pepper, then roast in the oven for 14 minutes, turning halfway.

While the midget trees are roasting, toast the almonds in a dry frying pan over a medium heat until browned and smelling nutty, then allow to cool and roughly chop.

Make the Romanesco sauce by adding three-quarters of the almonds into a small food processor along with the roasted red pepper, remaining paprika, olive oil, garlic and a good pinch of salt and pepper. Blitz until smooth, adding the vinegar to taste.

Drop the gnocchi into the pan of boiling water and cook according to packet instructions. Drain, then put back in the pan and spoon in the sauce. Mix together so that the sauce heats through.

Spoon onto a plate, place the baked broccoli on top and scatter over the remaining almonds. Grate over some cheese, if using.

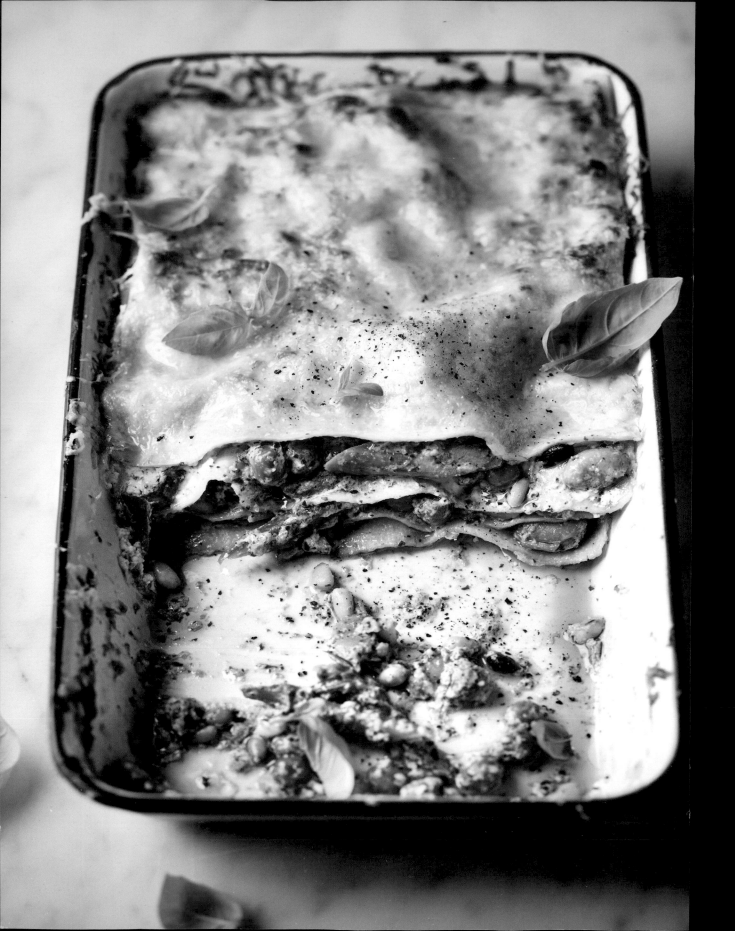

My lovely lasagne

LONGER RECIPE

Ingredients

1 tbsp olive oil
1 clove garlic
100g asparagus, each cut
  into three pieces
100g frozen peas
100g frozen broad beans
100g pesto
zest of 1 lemon
150g mascarpone
50g vegetarian hard cheese,
  finely grated
salt and pepper
6 lasagne sheets
4 tbsp milk
green salad, to serve

Method

Preheat the oven to 180°C (fan 160°C, gas mark 4). Grab yourself a smallish ovenproof dish.

Heat the olive oil in a frying pan over a medium heat. Crush in the garlic clove and tip in the asparagus. Cook for 2 minutes, then stir in the frozen peas and broad beans. Cook for another minute until the peas and broad beans have thawed.

Take the pan off the heat and chuck the greens into a bowl. Mix through the pesto, lemon zest, 100g mascarpone, half the grated cheese and some salt and pepper.

Spoon a third of the mix into the ovenproof dish, then top with two sheets of lasagne. Repeat the process until all the filling and pasta are used up. For the final layer, mix the remaining mascarpone with the milk. Pour this over the top of the pasta sheets and sprinkle over the remaining hard cheese.

Bake for 35–40 minutes until the pasta has no resistance when you prick it with a fork. Leave to rest for 5 minutes before diving in. Serve with a green salad.

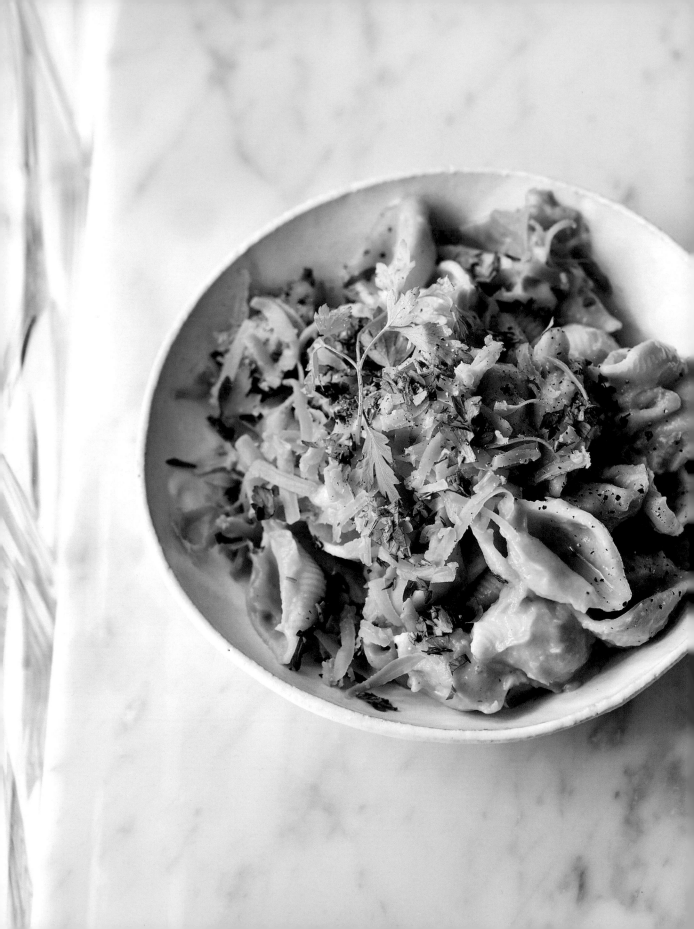

Joe's creamy dreamy butternut pasta

Ingredients

½ small butternut squash, peeled and chopped into small pieces

150g pasta shells

salt and pepper

1 clove garlic, peeled

100ml veg stock

2 tbsp double cream

½ tsp smoked paprika

big pinch of nutmeg

handful of parsley, roughly chopped, plus extra sprigs to garnish

30g red leicester cheese, grated

Method

Place two saucepans of water on to boil. Chuck the butternut squash pieces into one of the pans and cook for 8 minutes until soft. Drop the pasta shells into the other, season the water with salt, then cook for 1 minute less than packet instructions.

When the butternut squash is soft, drain it and tip into a blender along with the garlic clove, veg stock, cream, smoked paprika, nutmeg and a good pinch of salt and pepper. Blitz to a smooth creamy sauce.

Drain the pasta in a colander, tip back into the saucepan and stir through the butternut sauce and parsley.

Spoon into your bowl and top with the grated cheese and parsley sprigs.

MAKE AHEAD

Ingredients

salt
120g orzo pasta
1 courgette
1 tbsp parsley, chopped
zest and juice of 1 lemon
1–1½ tbsp harissa paste
1 tbsp olive oil
50g feta, crumbled

Harissa orzo with courgette and feta

Method

Bring a saucepan of water to the boil. When boiling, season with salt, then drop in the orzo. Give the pasta a good stir, then cook for 1 minute less than packet instructions.

While the pasta is cooking, use a peeler to peel the courgette into long ribbons. Save the seeded core for another time. Toss the courgette ribbons in the parsley, lemon zest and juice and a generous pinch of salt.

Drain the pasta into a colander, saving half a mugful of pasta water. Tip the pasta back into the pan and stir through the harissa and olive oil. Splash in a little pasta water, adding enough to make the orzo shiny. Stir through the feta.

Tip the pasta into a bowl. Top with the ribbons of courgette, spooning over the lemon juice and parsley.

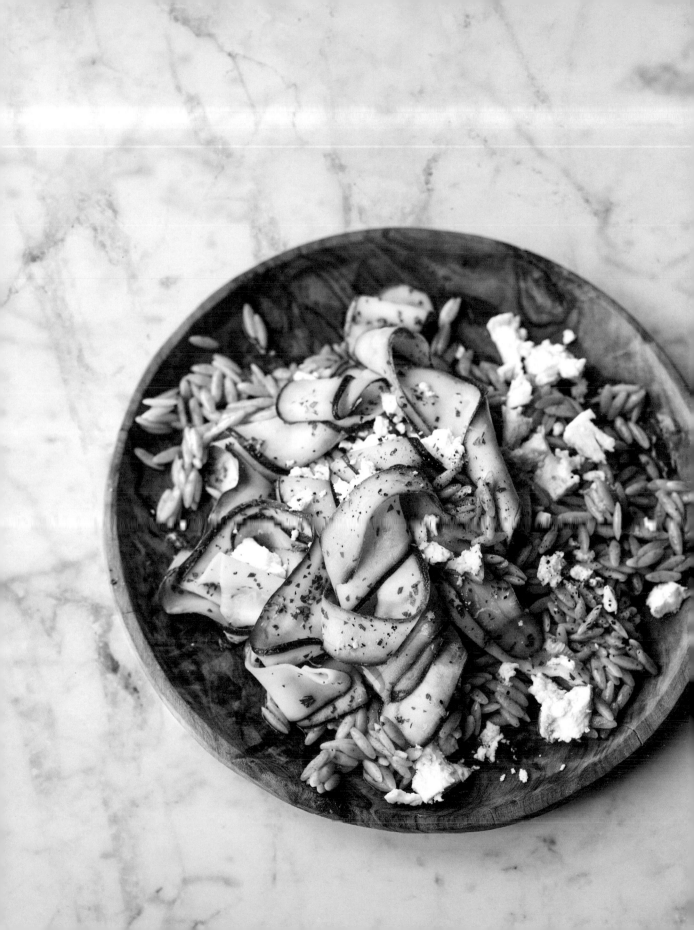

**SERVES
1**

Courgette and chilli carbonara

Ingredients

salt and black pepper
130g penne
1 large courgette
1 tbsp olive oil
1 red chilli, de-seeded and
  finely chopped
30g vegetarian hard cheese
2 egg yolks
2 tbsp single cream

Method

Bring a saucepan of water to the boil. Season with salt.

Drop the penne into the water, give it a good stir so the pasta doesn't stick together, then cook for 1 minute less than packet instructions.

Halve the courgette lengthways then use a teaspoon to scrape out the fluffy seeded core. Cut into half-moon slices.

Put the oil in a large frying pan over a medium to high heat. Chuck in the courgette with a pinch of salt, fry for 6 minutes or until softened and charred in places, then stir in the chilli and cook for 1 minute more.

While the courgette is cooking, finely grate the cheese. Using a fork, whisk together the egg yolks, single cream and cheese in a jug.

Drain the pasta, saving a mugful of the pasta water, then drop the pasta into the frying pan along with the courgette. Give it a good stir, then take off the heat and pour in the creamy egg mixture, along with a splash of saved pasta water.

Toss everything together. You want the pasta to be coated in a shiny silky sauce. If it looks a bit thick, stir in more of the pasta water. If you've added a little too much water, put the pan back on the lowest heat and cook for a minute.

Tip into a bowl, crack over some black pepper and eat straight away.

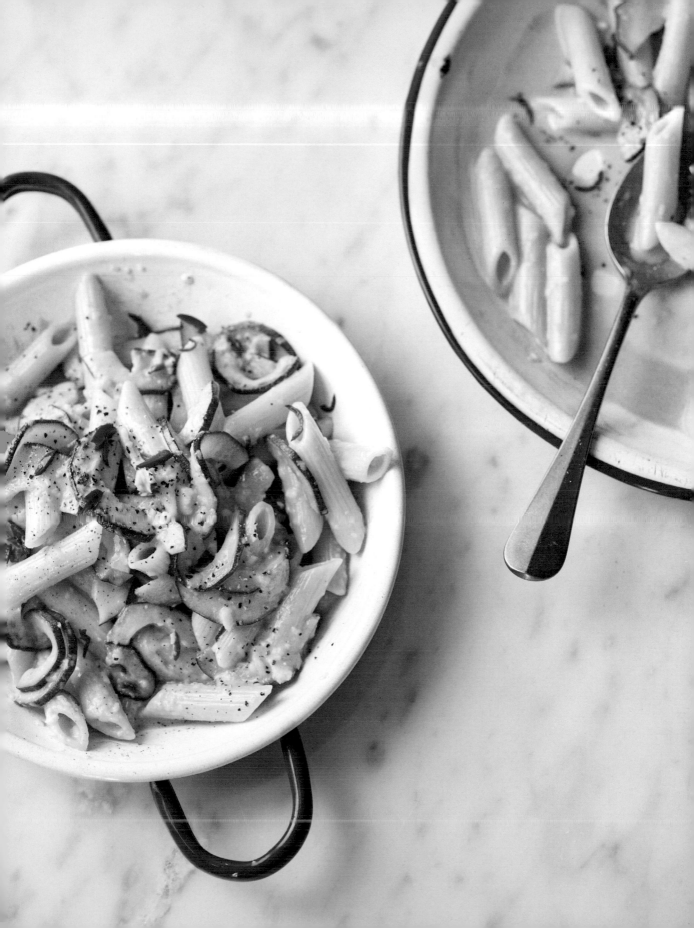

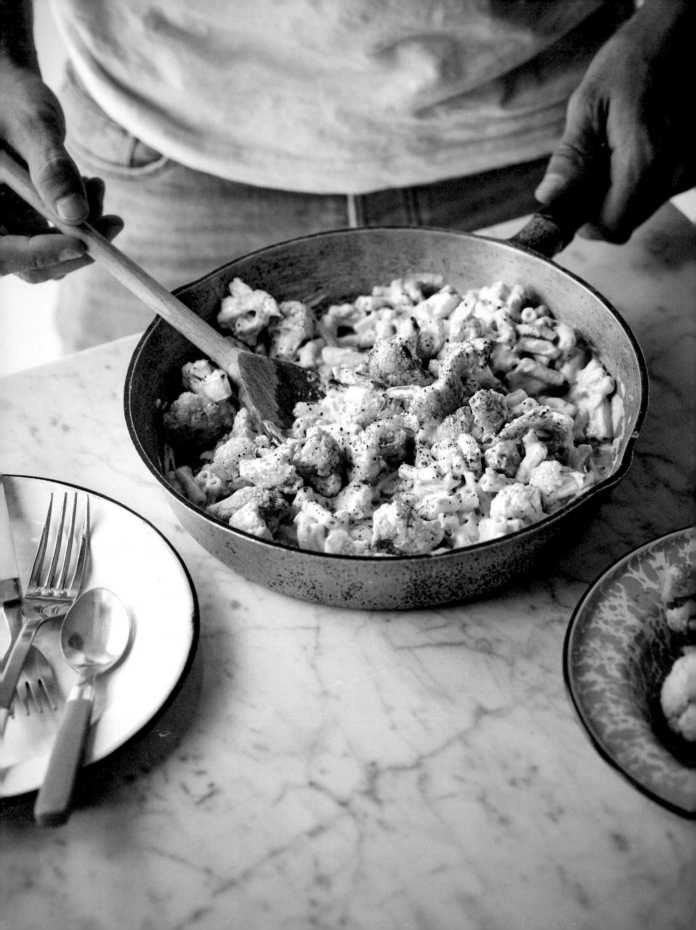

SERVES 1 **VE**

Vegan cauliflower mac 'n' cheese

LONGER RECIPE

Ingredients

50g cashew nuts
½ small head of cauliflower,
   florets only
2 tbsp olive oil
1 tsp smoked paprika
salt and black pepper
100g macaroni
½ tsp dijon mustard
1 small clove garlic, peeled
big pinch of ground turmeric
1–2 tbsp nutritional yeast
   (depending on how 'cheesy'
   you like it)

Method

Preheat your grill to maximum and bring a kettle of water to the boil.

Tip the cashews into a blender and pour 150ml boiling water over the top. Leave to soak for 5 minutes. Pour the rest of the boiling water into a saucepan for the pasta.

Put the cauliflower florets on a flat roasting sheet and mix with 1 tablespoon of the olive oil, ½ teaspoon smoked paprika and a good pinch of salt and pepper. Whack under the grill for 15 minutes, turning halfway.

While the cauliflower is cooking, salt the water in the saucepan then drop in the macaroni. Cook for 1 minute less than packet instructions.

To make your vegan cheese sauce, come back to your cashews. Add the remaining olive oil, paprika, mustard, garlic, turmeric and nutritional yeast to the blender. Blitz the sauce until smooth and season to taste. Don't worry if it looks runny at this point, it will thicken as it hits the pasta!

Drain the pasta and put it back in the saucepan. Mix through the grilled cauliflower and the vegan cheese sauce, then put back on the hob for 1 minute to heat through. Spoon into a bowl and crack over some more black pepper to serve.

Spinach and ricotta tortellini with salsa verde

Ingredients

handful of parsley
1 small clove garlic
½ tbsp capers
½ tsp dijon mustard
1½ tbsp olive oil
salt and pepper
squeeze of lemon juice
**250g spinach and ricotta
  tortellini**
**30g vegetarian hard cheese,
  finely grated**

Method

Bring a large saucepan of water to the boil.

Meanwhile, make the salsa verde. Chop the parsley, garlic and capers as finely as you can. Scrape into a bowl and, using a fork, whisk in the dijon mustard and olive oil. Season with salt and pepper and lemon juice to taste.

Season the boiling water with a little salt then drop in the tortellini. Cook according to packet instructions then drain into a colander. Shake off any excess water then put the pasta back into the pan and stir through the salsa verde. Shake everything together so each piece gets coated in the sauce.

Pile into a bowl and sprinkle over the grated cheese.

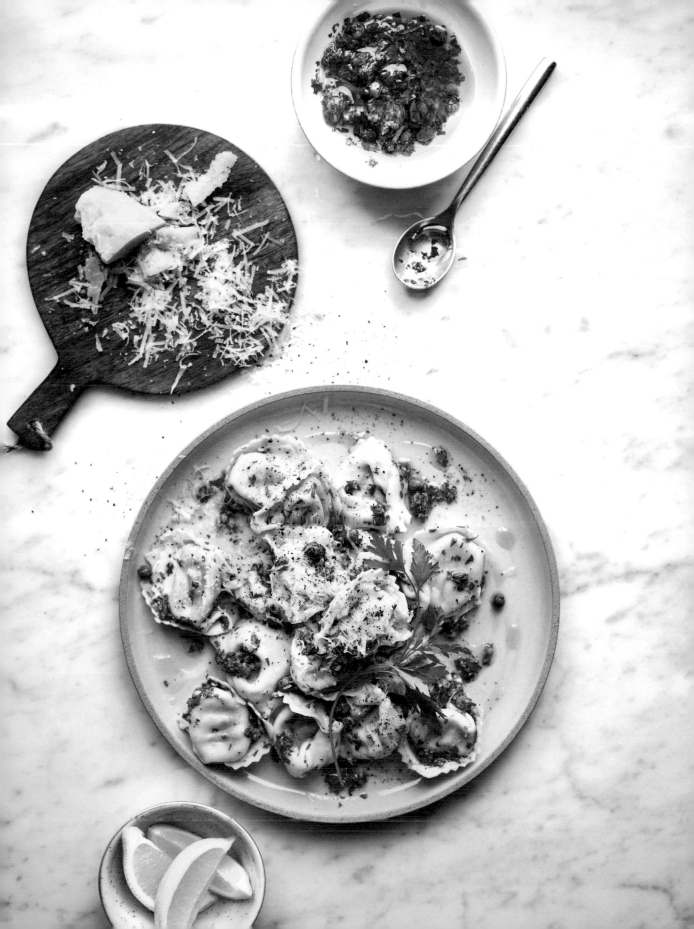

**SERVES
1**

Moroccan spiced giant couscous with halloumi

MAKE AHEAD
Add the halloumi just before serving.

Ingredients

**salt and black pepper
100g giant couscous
2 carrots, peeled
handful of mint leaves
handful of parsley
2 dried apricots
1 tbsp olive oil
½ tsp smoked paprika
pinch of ground cinnamon
6 thin slices of halloumi**

Method

Bring a saucepan of water to the boil. Season with a little salt. Drop in the giant couscous, then cook for 1 minute less than packet instructions.

Meanwhile peel the carrots lengthways into long ribbons and put into a bowl. Roughly chop the mint leaves, parsley and dried apricots. Add to the bowl with the carrots. Pour in the olive oil, then add the paprika, cinnamon and a good pinch of salt and pepper. Toss to combine, then set aside.

Drain the giant couscous into a sieve, then rinse under cold water. Shake off any excess water, then tip the couscous into the bowl with the carrots and give everything a good stir. Tip onto a plate.

Place a dry non-stick frying pan over a high heat. Add the halloumi slices and fry for 2 minutes on each side until golden brown. Place the halloumi on top of the giant couscous and get stuck in.

 **JOE'S
TOP TIP** | Rinsing the couscous helps to get rid of any excess starch and stops it from being claggy.

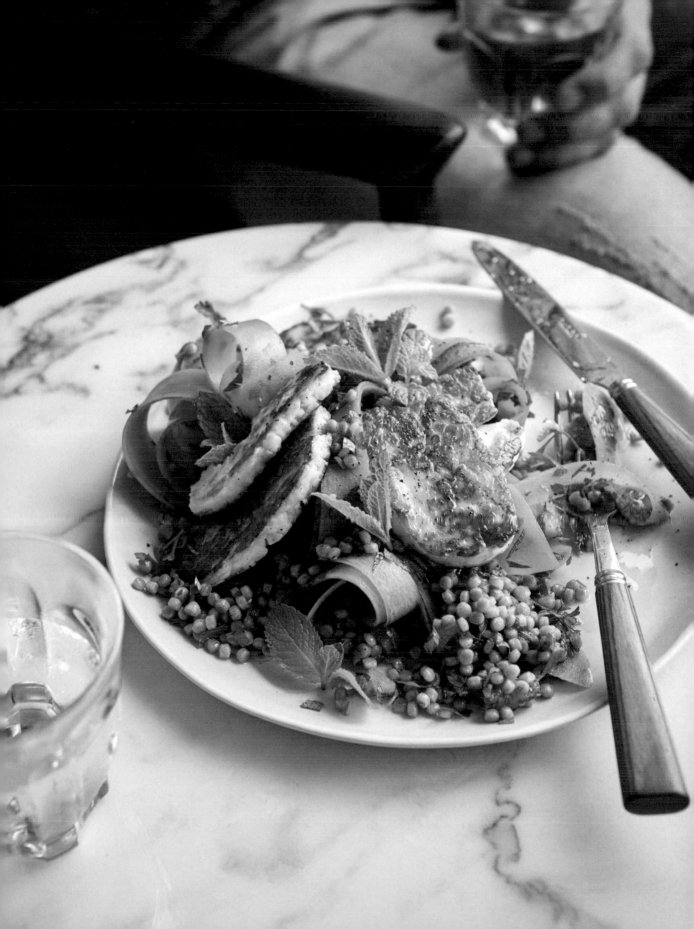

5-a-day vegetable paella

LONGER RECIPE

Ingredients

2 tbsp coconut oil
1 fennel bulb, sliced
1 courgette, sliced into
  half-moons
2 small mixed colour peppers,
  sliced – I like red and yellow
salt and pepper
2 cloves garlic, crushed
1½ tsp smoked paprika
6 sundried tomatoes,
  roughly chopped
180g paella or arborio
  rice
glass of white wine
800ml veg stock
100g chargrilled artichokes
  (from a pack or jarred),
  roughly chopped
8 pitted green olives, halved
handful of parsley leaves,
  roughly chopped
50g toasted flaked almonds
½ lemon, cut into wedges

Method

Melt the coconut oil in a large frying pan over a medium heat.

Tip in the sliced fennel, courgette and peppers along with some salt and pepper. Cook for 6–8 minutes until mostly softened.

Stir in the garlic, smoked paprika and sundried tomatoes. Cook for 1 minute until it smells fragrant, then tip in the rice. Give everything a good stir, then slug in the white wine. When the wine has bubbled off, pour in the veg stock.

Simmer the paella, stirring occasionally so it doesn't stick to the bottom of the pan, until most of the stock has been absorbed by the rice. This usually takes 20 minutes.

Stir in the artichokes and olives. Cook for a couple more minutes, season to taste, then scatter over the parsley and flaked almonds and nestle in the lemon wedges. Serve straight out of the pan.

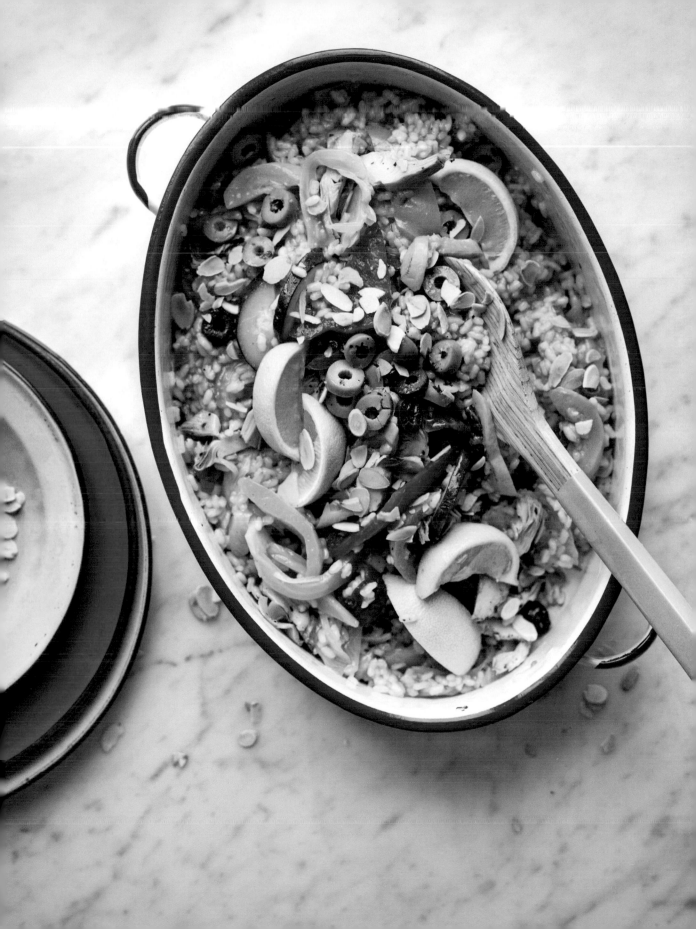

Ginger and garlic rice bowl

SERVES 1

Ingredients

knob of fresh ginger, peeled
1 small clove garlic
1 small shallot, finely chopped
1 tsp honey
juice of ½ lemon
2½ tbsp olive oil
salt and pepper
30g cashew nuts
1 egg – optional
150g pre-cooked wholegrain
  rice
½ avocado, de-stoned
  and sliced
½ cucumber, peeled
  lengthways, seedy core
  discarded
small handful of coriander,
  roughly chopped

Method

Grate the ginger and garlic into a small bowl. Add the shallot, honey, lemon juice and 2 tablespoons of the olive oil. Whisk the dressing together, then season to taste, adding more ginger and lemon juice if you want.

Toast the cashew nuts in a dry small frying pan over a medium heat, then allow to cool and roughly chop.

If you're serving with an egg, put the pan back on the heat and pour in the remaining oil. Crack in the egg and fry to your liking.

While the egg is cooking, ping the rice in the microwave according to packet instructions.

Tip into your serving bowl and while hot, stir in the ginger and garlic dressing. Lay the avocado slices and cucumber ribbons in the bowl. Slide on the fried egg, if using, then scatter over the coriander and cashew nuts.

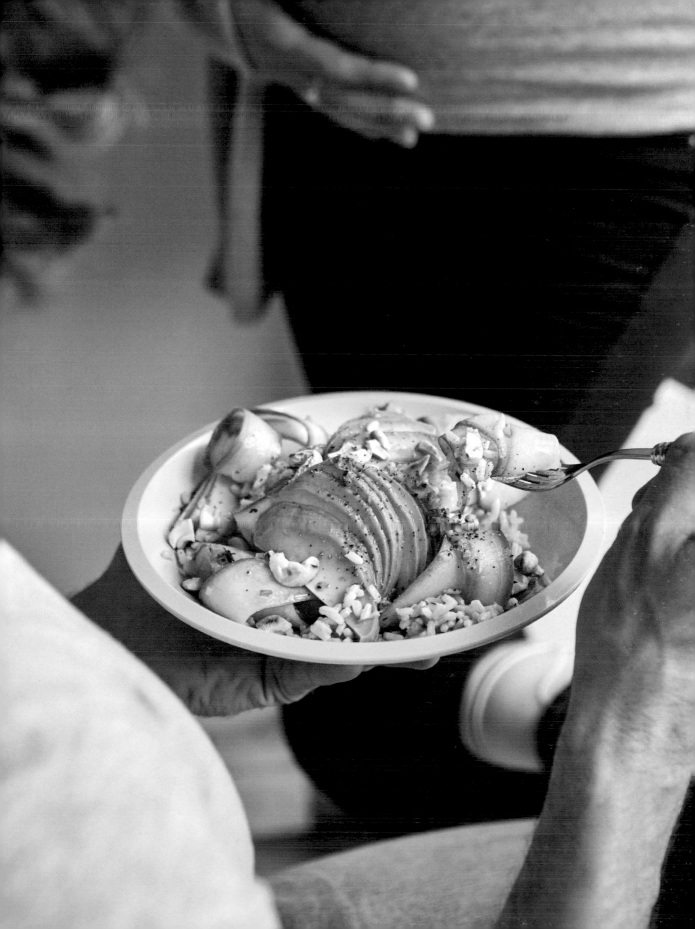

Garlicky mushrooms on cheesy polenta

Ingredients

2 tbsp butter

200g mushrooms of your
 choice, sliced

1 fat clove garlic, finely
 chopped

salt and pepper

300ml veg stock

70g quick-cook polenta

50g vegetarian hard cheese,
 finely grated

handful of parsley, half
 chopped, half left as sprigs

Method

Melt half the butter in a frying pan over a high heat.
Tip the mushrooms into the pan along with the garlic and
a pinch of salt and pepper. Fry for 5 minutes, until all the
water has come out of the mushrooms and they have turned
golden. Turn down the heat to low and keep warm.

Pour the stock into a saucepan over a medium heat and
bring to the boil. Grab a whisk.

When the stock starts to bubble, pour the polenta into
the stock in a steady stream, whisking all the time. Keep
whisking and cooking for 5 minutes until the polenta
has cooked through and thickened.

Whisk in the remaining butter and cheese along with
some salt and pepper and the chopped parsley. Spoon
the polenta into a bowl, top with the garlicky mushrooms
and top with the parsley sprigs.

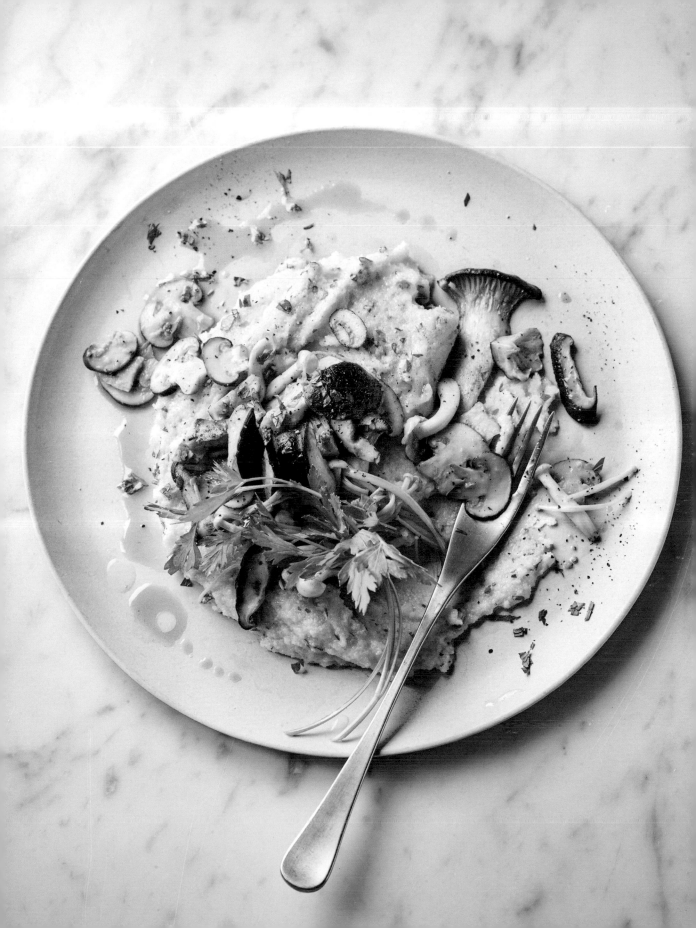

Grilled cheesy gnocchi with leeks and mustard

Ingredients

- 1 tbsp coconut oil
- 2 leeks, trimmed and finely sliced
- salt
- 200g gnocchi
- 100ml veg stock
- 50ml double cream
- 1 tsp wholegrain mustard
- 50g mature cheddar, grated

Method

Preheat your grill to maximum. Bring a kettle of water to the boil.

Melt the coconut oil in a frying pan over a medium heat. Add the leeks and a pinch of salt. Fry for 5 minutes until softened.

Meanwhile, pour the boiling water into a saucepan. Drop in the gnocchi and cook according to packet instructions, then drain into a colander. Shake off any excess water, then tip the gnocchi into a small ovenproof dish. Spoon the leeks on top of the gnocchi.

Mix the veg stock with the double cream and mustard. Pour this over the top of the gnocchi, then scatter with the cheese. Grill until bubbling, then allow the gnocchi to rest for a few minutes before eating.

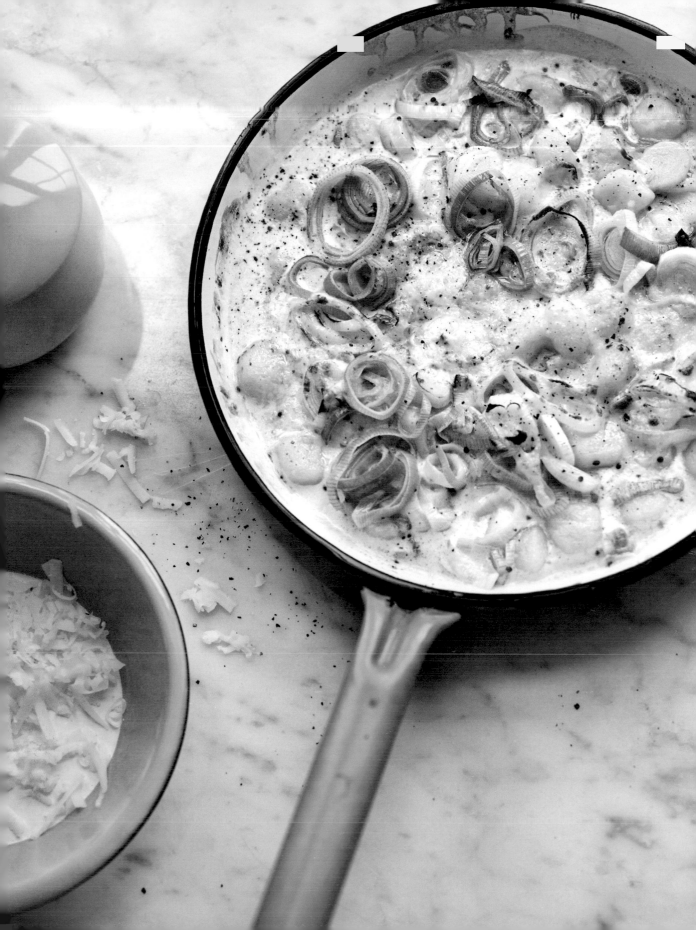

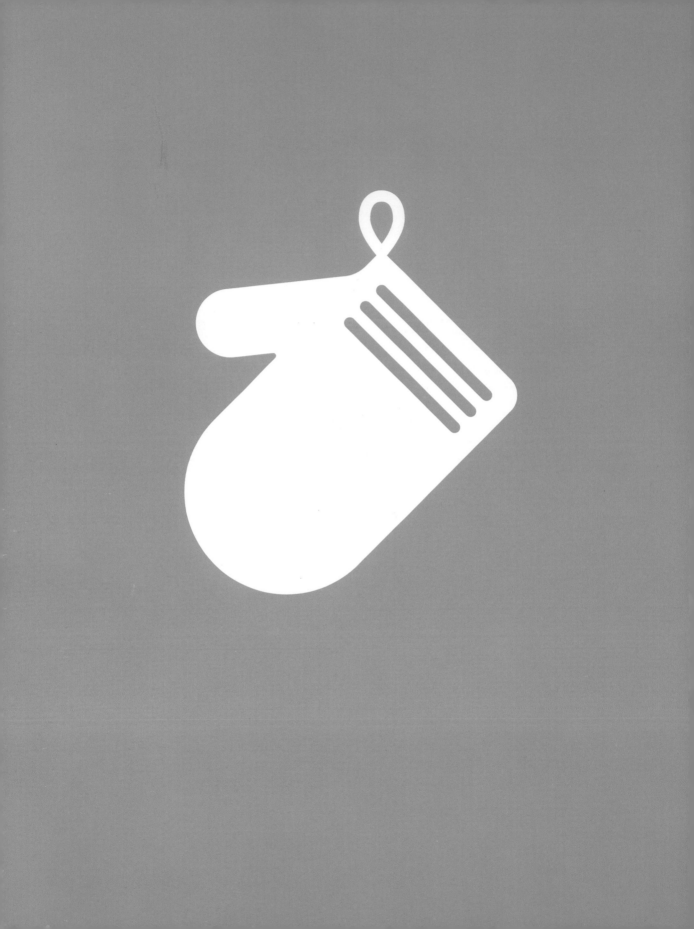

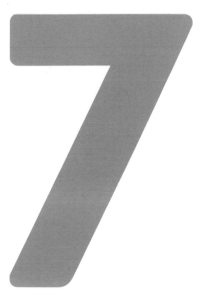

7

BAKES AND ROASTS

SERVES 1

Baked Mediterranean feta

Ingredients

100g feta
200g passata
1 clove garlic, crushed
1 tsp balsamic vinegar
½ tsp dried oregano
zest of 1 lemon
salt and pepper
8–10 pitted mixed olives,
  halved
drizzle of olive oil
a few basil leaves
crusty bread – like ciabatta,
  to serve

Method

Preheat the oven to 200°C (fan 180°C, gas mark 6).

Place the feta in a small ovenproof dish. Add the passata to a medium bowl along with the crushed garlic, balsamic vinegar, oregano, lemon zest and a good pinch of salt and pepper. Stir together then pour the sauce over the feta. Scatter over the olives, then roast for 14 minutes.

When baked, drizzle with a little olive oil and scatter over the basil leaves. Serve straight out of the ovenproof dish with bread.

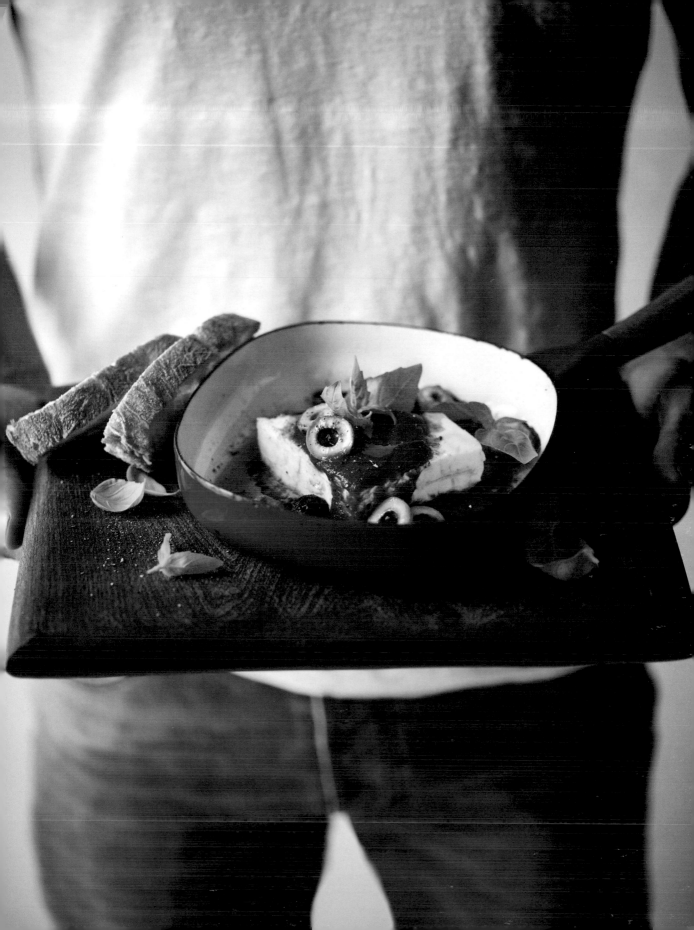

**LONGER RECIPE
MAKE AHEAD**
Enjoy hot or cold.

Ingredients

350g frozen spinach
3 cloves garlic, crushed
3 eggs
250g jarred roasted red
   peppers, drained and
   chopped
200g feta cheese, crumbled
large handful of
   parsley, chopped
½ tsp dried chilli flakes
zest and juice of 1 lemon
1 pack filo pastry (12 sheets)
75g melted butter
2 tbsp sesame seeds
salt and pepper
green salad, to serve

Roasted red pepper and feta filo-tastic

Method

Preheat the oven to 200°C (fan 180°C, gas mark 6) and bring a kettle of water to the boil.

Put the frozen spinach in a bowl. Pour over the boiling water and leave for a couple of minutes to defrost.

Meanwhile, place the garlic in a separate bowl, crack in the eggs and stir through the remaining ingredients apart from the pastry, butter and sesame seeds.

Drain the spinach and use your hands to squeeze out as much water as possible, then add to the bowl with the other ingredients. Beat everything together with a wooden spoon to combine, then season with salt and pepper.

Line a flat baking sheet with a piece of baking parchment. Unravel the filo pastry from its packet, then keep the sheets under a damp tea towel to stop them from drying out.

Place one sheet of filo on the baking parchment, brush all over with melted butter, then sprinkle over a few sesame seeds. Slap another on top at a slightly different angle, then repeat this process until you've used up all the pastry, saving a little butter and sesame seeds for the top of the tart. When you have used up all of the pastry you will have created a wonky star shape.

Spoon the filling into the centre of your pastry star. Flatten it into a rough circle with the back of your spoon, then gather in the pastry from around the edges so you are left with an enclosed pie with an exposed centre.

Brush the top of the pastry with the remaining butter and sprinkle over the remaining sesame seeds. Transfer to the oven for 25–30 minutes until the pastry is deep golden brown.

Resist the temptation to gobble down straight away and leave it to cool for 5 minutes, then cut into slices. Serve with a green salad.

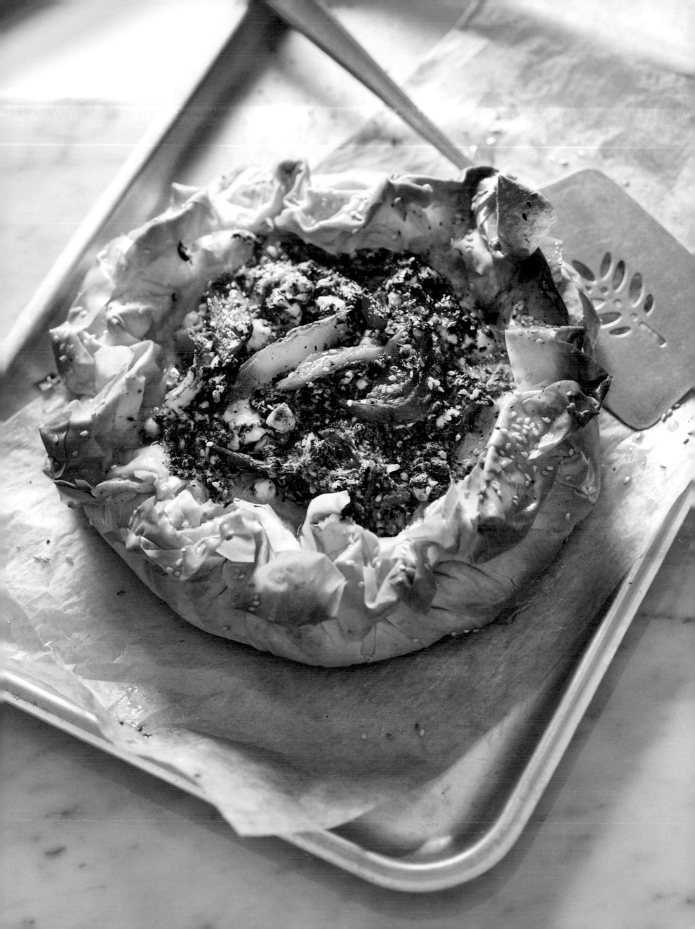

SERVES 2

Mediterranean vegetable puff pastry tart

Ingredients

1 sheet ready-rolled
  puff pastry
2 tbsp olive oil
1 red onion, finely sliced
1 courgette, finely sliced
2 mixed colour peppers,
  finely sliced
salt and pepper
2 cloves garlic
8 cherry tomatoes, halved
handful of basil leaves
4 spoonfuls of ricotta
zest of 1 lemon
pinch of dried chilli flakes
green salad, to serve

Method

Preheat the oven to 220°C (fan 200°C, gas mark 7).
Put a flat baking sheet in the oven to get hot.

Unravel the puff pastry, then use a sharp knife to score
a border 1cm away from the pastry edge, being careful not
to cut all the way through. This will encourage the sides to
rise. Put the pastry onto the hot baking sheet and cook for
15 minutes until deep golden brown and cooked through.

Meanwhile, heat the olive oil in a large frying pan over a
medium heat. Chuck in the sliced red onion, courgette
and peppers along with a good pinch of salt. Fry, stirring
regularly for 5 minutes until the veg have collapsed and
mostly softened. Crush the garlic cloves straight into the
pan and scrape in the tomatoes. Cook for a further 5 minutes
until the tomatoes have all burst. Season with salt and
pepper to taste, then stir through the basil leaves.

Slide the baked pastry case onto a board then pile the veg
in the centre. Don't worry if the whole thing has puffed up,
the veg will flatten it.

Dot over the ricotta, then scatter with lemon zest and
chilli flakes. Serve with a green salad.

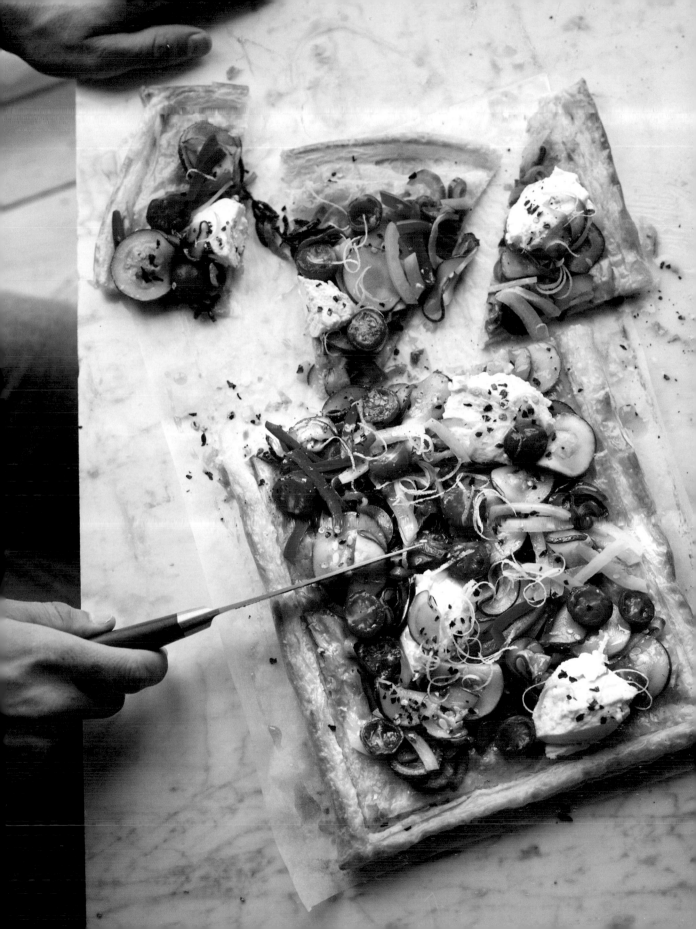

SERVES 2

Loaded sweet potato skins

LONGER RECIPE

Ingredients

1 large sweet potato, skin on
½ avocado, de-stoned
1 lime
4 cherry tomatoes, roughly chopped
salt and pepper
½ tbsp olive oil
200g black beans, drained and rinsed
2 spring onions, finely sliced
1 tsp fajita seasoning
1 clove garlic, finely chopped
30g cheddar, grated
hot sauce, to serve

Method

Preheat the oven to 220°C (fan 200°C, gas mark 7).

Cut the sweet potato in half and place it in a microwaveable bowl. Cover with cling film then zap on high for 8 minutes.

Meanwhile, make the guac. Scoop the avocado into a bowl, squeeze in juice of half the lime, then use your fork to roughly mash. Stir in the cherry tomatoes and season to taste.

Get the sweet potato out of the microwave, leave until cool enough to handle, then scoop out the flesh into a bowl. Place the skins on a flat roasting sheet, drizzle with the oil, then whack in the oven for 5 minutes to crisp up.

Meanwhile, mash the sweet potato flesh with a fork, then stir in the black beans, spring onion, fajita seasoning and garlic along with some salt and pepper. Finely slice the remaining half of lime.

Fill each crisp potato skin with the black bean mixture, piling high. Scatter over the cheddar, return to the oven and bake for 5 minutes until the cheese has melted and browned.

Serve with hot sauce, the guac and lime slices.

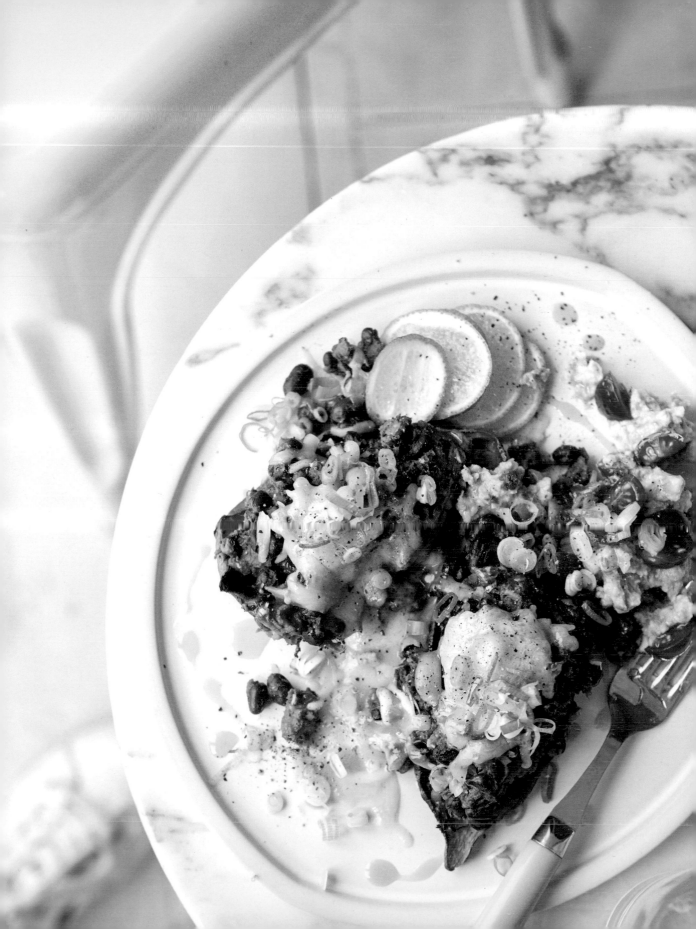

Veggie parmigiana

Ingredients

1½ tbsp olive oil
½ red onion, finely chopped
salt and black pepper
1 courgette, cut into chunky
   diagonal slices
½ aubergine, cut into
   half-moons
1 yellow pepper, cut into
   quarters
1 clove garlic, crushed
250g passata
½ tbsp red wine vinegar
a few basil leaves
½ ball of mozzarella (75g)
30g vegetarian hard cheese,
   finely grated
1 tbsp pine nuts
garlic bread and salad,
   to serve

Method

Preheat your grill to maximum. Tear a piece of tin foil to line the bottom of a grill pan or a flat baking sheet with a wire rack put on top.

Pour ½ tablespoon olive oil into a saucepan over a medium heat. Tip in the onion along with a pinch of salt. Cook for 5 minutes.

Keeping the veg separate, lay out the courgette, aubergine and yellow pepper on the rack in a single layer, then drizzle over the remaining oil along with some salt and pepper. Whack under the grill for 10 minutes until soft, turning halfway.

Stir the garlic into the onion pan and cook for 1 minute until it smells fragrant, then pour in your passata and red wine vinegar. Bubble the sauce away for 10 minutes. Take the pan off the heat, stir in the basil leaves and season to taste.

Now to build your parmigiana. Grab yourself a small ovenproof dish. Put all the aubergine slices at the bottom, then spoon over one-third of the sauce, then a third of the mozzarella and grated cheese. Repeat the process with the pepper, then the courgette. Scatter over the pine nuts then slide back under the grill for 8–10 minutes until the cheese is oozing, crisp and golden brown.

Let the parmigiana sit for 5 minutes, then gobble down with garlic bread and salad.

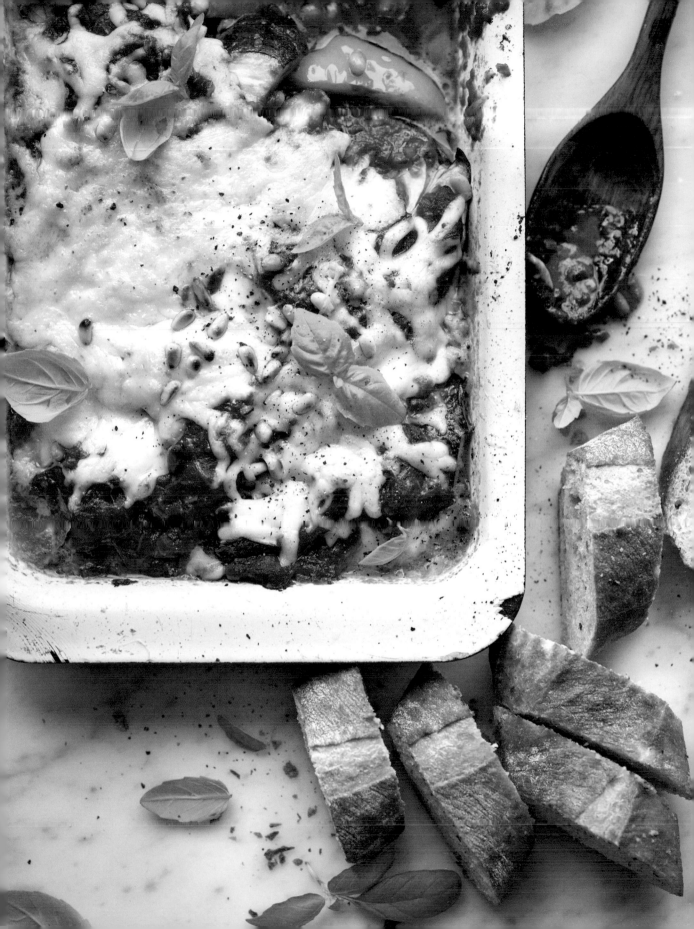

SERVES 1

Green couscous stuffed courgette

Ingredients

1 large courgette
2 tbsp olive oil, plus extra
  for drizzling
salt
50g couscous
small handful of mint leaves
small handful of parsley
  (stalks and all)
50g brie, sliced
1 spring onion, finely sliced
1 tbsp toasted pine nuts
rocket salad, to serve

Method

Preheat the oven to 220°C (fan 200°C/gas mark 7).
Bring a kettle of water to the boil.

Cut the courgette in half lengthways then use a spoon
to scrape out the middle. Put on a baking tray cut-side
down and drizzle with a little olive oil. Season with salt,
then roast for 10 minutes.

Meanwhile, pour 100ml boiling water over the couscous in
a bowl. Cover with a plate or some cling film and leave to
steam for a few minutes. While it is steaming, blitz the mint,
parsley and remaining olive oil in a small food processor
to a herby paste. Add a splash of water if it looks too thick
– you want the consistency of pesto.

Come back to the couscous. Use a fork to fluff up the
grains, then mix through your herby paste to turn it
bright green.

Take the courgette out of the oven and heat the grill
to maximum. Flip the courgettes over and stuff with
the couscous mixture, then lay over the slices of brie.
Slide back under the grill and cook for 2–3 minutes
until the cheese is bubbling.

Transfer to a plate, scatter over the spring onion and
toasted pine nuts. Serve with a rocket salad.

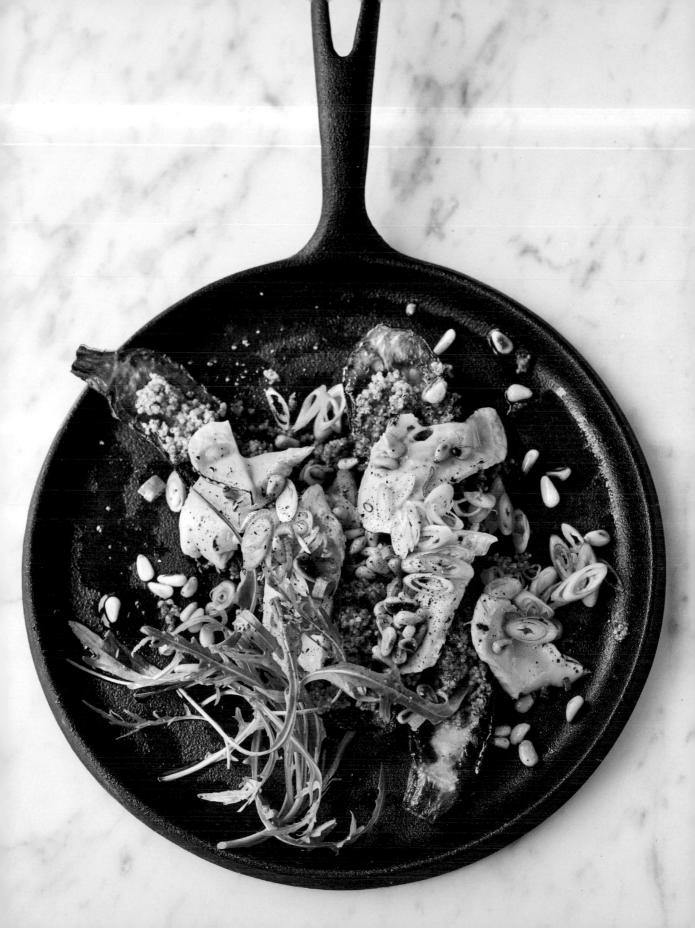

Curried root vegetable filo pie

LONGER RECIPE

Ingredients

40g butter
1 heaped tsp garlic–ginger
   paste
1 tbsp curry powder
1 tsp dried chilli flakes
1 medium carrot, peeled and
   cut into chunks
1 medium parsnip, peeled
   and cut into chunks
1 medium sweet potato,
   peeled and cut into chunks
1 x 400ml tin of
   coconut milk
100ml veg stock
1 tbsp soy sauce
2 tbsp cashew butter
2 large handfuls of kale,
   stalks removed
½ pack filo pastry (6 sheets)
1 tbsp nigella (black onion)
   seeds

Method

Preheat the oven to 220°C (fan 200°C, gas mark 7).

Melt 1 tablespoon of the butter in a high-sided ovenproof frying pan over a medium heat. Stir in the garlic–ginger paste, curry powder, chilli flakes, chopped carrot, parsnip and sweet potato. Cook for 2 minutes, giving everything a good stir, then pour in the coconut milk and veg stock.

Simmer for 15 minutes until the vegetables are practically soft, then stir in the soy sauce, cashew butter and kale. When the kale has wilted, take the pan off the heat.

Melt the remaining butter in the microwave. Lay the pastry sheets out. Brush each one with the melted butter and scatter over the nigella seeds. Take a sheet of filo and roughly crumple it in your hand.

Place the crumpled sheet on top of the frying pan then repeat with the remaining filo sheets until the curried vegetables are completely covered.

Whack the pie in the oven for 15–20 minutes until the pastry is deep golden brown and crisp.

Leave to rest for 5 minutes before serving.

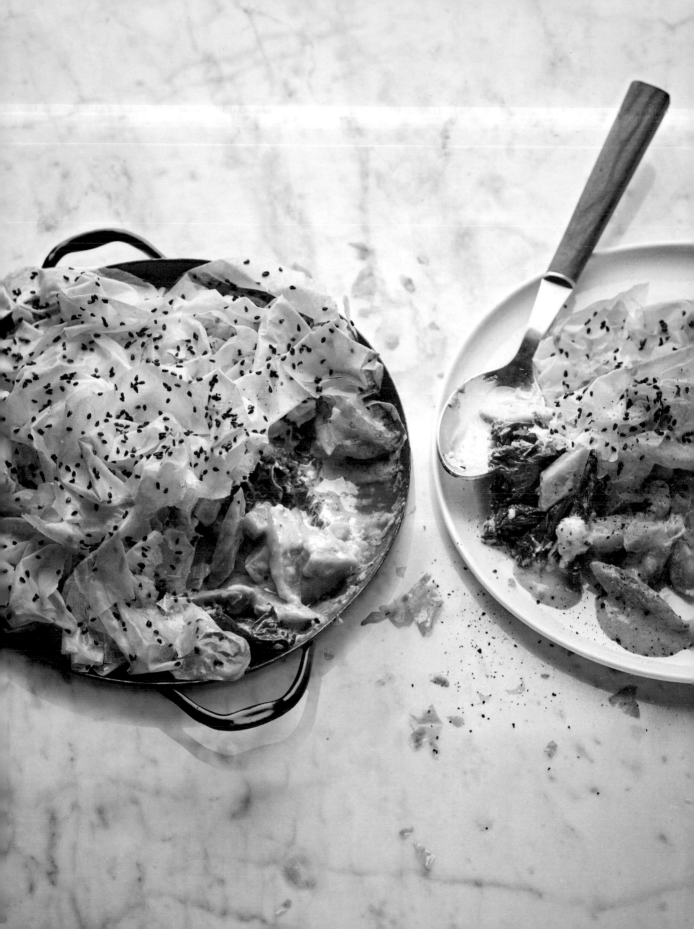

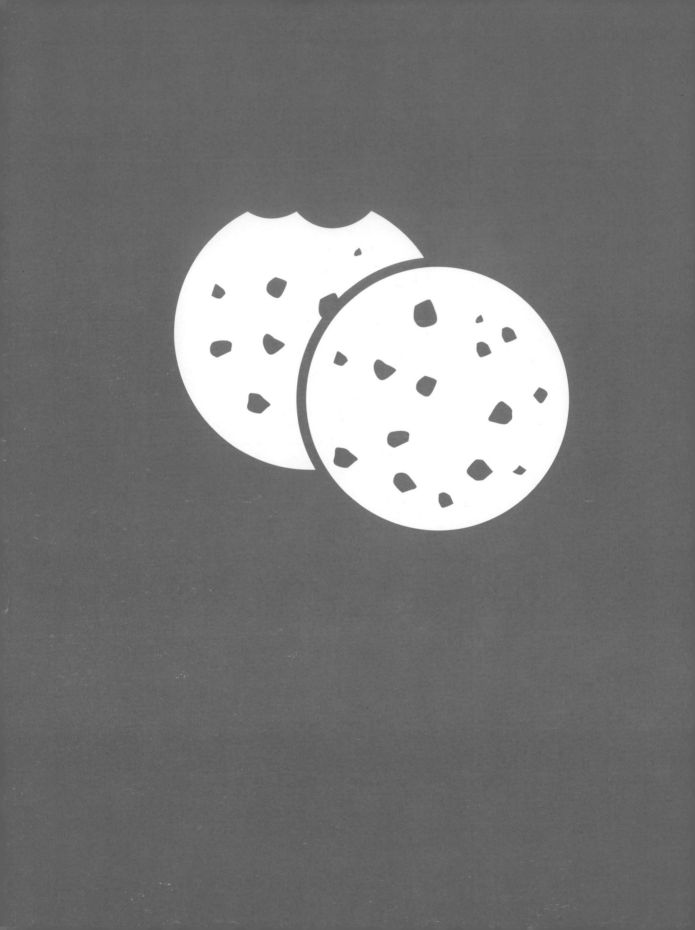

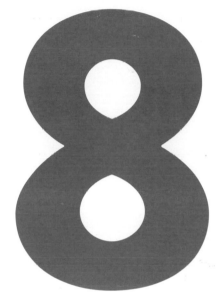

8

SNACKS AND SWEET TREATS

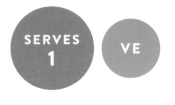

SERVES 1 **VE**

MAKE AHEAD

Ingredients

120g shelled frozen edamame beans
1 tsp sesame oil
1 tsp soy sauce
1 tsp sesame seeds

Sesame and soy edamame

Method

Bring a small saucepan of water to the boil. Drop in the edamame beans and cook for 3–4 minutes until tender, then drain into a colander and shake dry.

Heat the sesame oil in a frying pan. Chuck in the edamame and fry until blistered in places – a little bit of colour adds loads of flavour. Pour in the soy sauce and the sesame seeds.

Give the pan a good toss so that every bean gets nicely seasoned then tip into a bowl. Great eaten hot or cold. (Pictured overleaf.)

SERVES 1 **VE**

MAKE AHEAD
Keep in an airtight container for up to 1 day.

Ingredients

½ tbsp coconut oil
25g popping corn kernels
¼ tsp smoked paprika
salt

Paprika popcorn

Method

Find a sturdy lidded saucepan. Melt the coconut oil in the saucepan over a medium heat, then chuck in the popping corn kernels.

Put on the lid then let the kernels do their thing. You will hear when they start to pop. Shake the pan occasionally to encourage more to pop but don't take off the lid.

When the time between each pop slows to 2–3 seconds, take the pan off the heat.

Leave to settle for a minute, then sprinkle in the smoked paprika along with a good pinch of salt. Toss the popcorn so each piece gets coated in paprika, then tip into a bowl. Movie night on. (Pictured overleaf.)

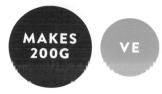

MAKES
200G

VE

MAKE AHEAD
Keep in an airtight container
for up to 1 week.

Ingredients

100g raw cashew nuts
100g blanched almonds
1 tbsp hot sauce – I like Sriracha
½ tsp maple syrup
1 tsp olive oil
salt

MAKES
16

MAKE AHEAD
Keep in an airtight container
for up to 1 week.

GOOD TO FREEZE
Bake from frozen, adding an extra
5 minutes to the cooking time.

Ingredients

1 pack ready-rolled puff pastry
1 tbsp Marmite
100g mature cheddar,
  finely grated
flour, for rolling

Joe's hot 'n' saucy nuts

Method

Preheat the oven to 190°C (fan 170°C, gas mark 5).
Line a flat baking sheet with a piece of baking parchment.

Mix all of the ingredients together, then tip onto the
baking sheet and spread out into a single layer so that
they cook evenly. Sprinkle with salt.

Roast in the oven for 8–12 minutes until the nuts are
lightly caramelized. (Pictured overleaf.)

Cheddar and Marmite straws

Method

Preheat the oven to 220°C (fan 200°C, gas mark 7).

Unravel the puff pastry onto a lightly floured surface. Cut the
parchment it came with in half and use to line two baking sheets.

Put the Marmite into a small bowl and zap in the microwave for
15 seconds so that it goes a bit runny. Use a spoon to drizzle it all
over the sheet of pastry. Scatter with three-quarters of the cheddar.

Fold the pastry in half like a book, then re-roll it out into a rectangle
with the thickness of a £1 coin. Using a sharp knife, cut the pastry
into 2cm strips along the shortest side, then use your fingers to
twizzle each strip 3–4 times into a corkscrew-shaped cheese straw.

Place the straws onto your lined baking sheets, sprinkle over the
remaining cheese and bake for 12–15 minutes, checking halfway
and turning the tray if some are becoming browner than others,
until cooked through and golden brown. (Pictured overleaf.)

JOE'S
TOP TIP

If you are a Marmite hater, spread the pastry
with 1 tablespoon of dijon mustard (there's
no need to heat it first).

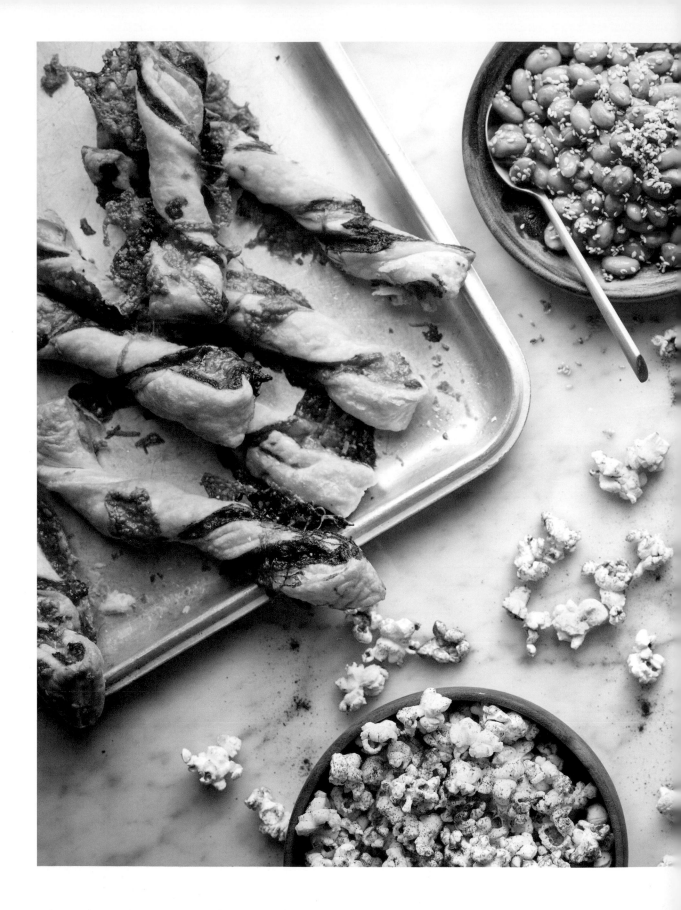

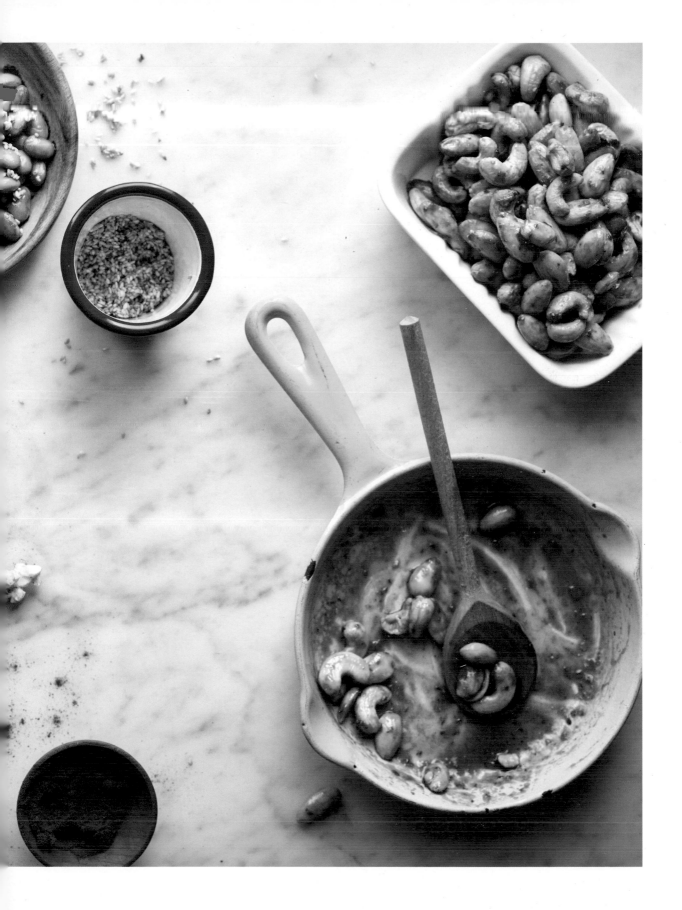

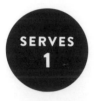

SERVES
1

Watermelon, feta and mint stacks

Ingredients

120g watermelon
30g feta
handful of mint leaves
pinch of dried chilli flakes
black pepper

Method

Cut away the skin from the watermelon if it has it on, then cut into squares. Cut the feta into smaller cubes to go on top.

Place a mint leaf on top of each cube of feta then sprinkle over a few chilli flakes and a crack of black pepper. Banging.

SERVES 1

Strawberry, ricotta and pumpkin seed toast

Ingredients

½ tbsp pumpkin seeds
salt
4 strawberries
1 slice of sourdough
1 spoonful of ricotta cheese
drizzle of honey

Method

Put the pumpkin seeds in a dry frying pan over a medium heat. Toast until they pop, then take off the heat and season with a little salt.

Remove the stalks from the strawberries and slice.

Toast your bread, then spread over the ricotta. Place the strawberries on top. Drizzle over a little honey, then top with the pumpkin seeds.

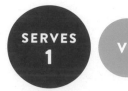

SERVES 1

VE

LONGER RECIPE

Ingredients

1 large sweet potato, skin on
1 tbsp coconut oil
½ tsp smoked paprika
salt and pepper
1 ripe avocado, de-stoned
4 cherry tomatoes, roughly
  chopped
2 tbsp coriander, roughly
  chopped
juice of ½ lime

Sweet potato fries and guacamole

Method

Preheat the oven to 220°C (fan 200°C, gas mark 7).

Scrub and wash your sweet potato to get rid of any dirt, then cut the sweet potato into fries about 1cm thick.

Melt the coconut oil in a large bowl in the microwave, then stir in the smoked paprika along with a generous pinch of salt and pepper. Chuck in the sweet potato fries and use your hands to toss them in the spiced oil.

Tip the sweet potato onto a large flat baking sheet and separate them out so they are in a single layer and not overcrowded. Roast for 20–25 minutes until crisp.

While the fries are roasting, scoop the avocado into a bowl and roughly mash with a fork. Stir in the cherry tomatoes, chopped coriander, lime juice, and salt and pepper to taste.

Serve the fries hot with the guacamole.

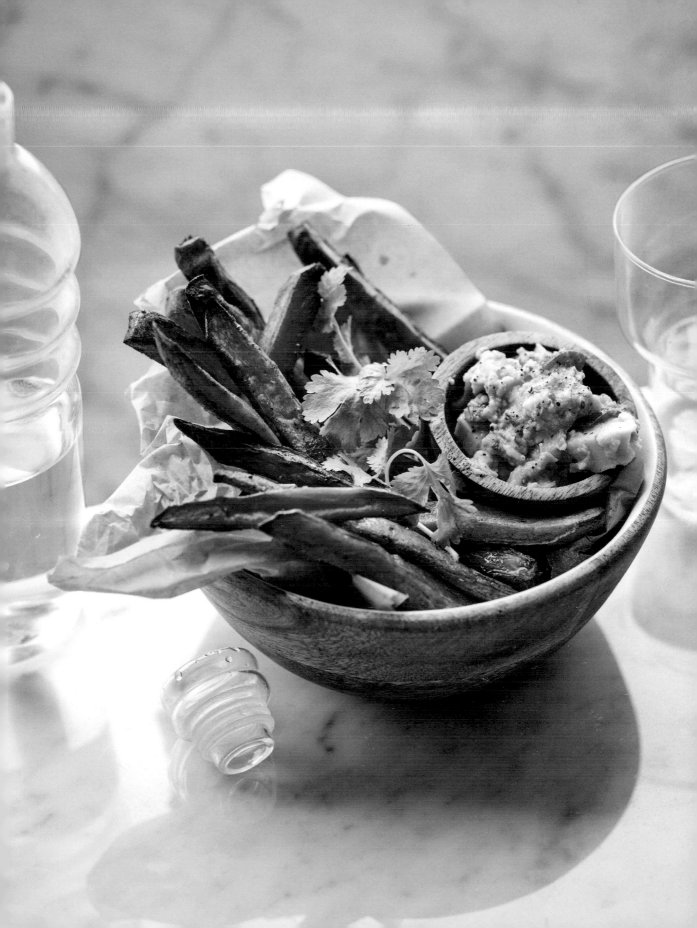

Popcorn cauliflower with chipotle mayo

LONGER RECIPE

Ingredients

1 tbsp olive oil

20g vegetarian hard cheese, finely grated

½ tsp mustard powder

good pinch of garlic powder – optional

salt and pepper

150g cauliflower, florets only

1 tsp chipotle paste

1 tbsp mayo

Method

Preheat the oven to 220°C (fan 200°C, gas mark 7). Tear some tin foil and line the bottom of a flat baking sheet.

Mix the olive oil, three-quarters of the grated cheese, the mustard powder and garlic powder, if using, in a bowl along with a generous pinch of salt and pepper. Add the cauliflower florets and toss to combine, so that each piece of cauliflower gets coated in the mixture.

Tip the cauliflower onto the baking sheet. Separate the florets so that they are in a single layer and aren't overcrowded. Roast for 15 minutes, then sprinkle on the rest of the cheese and roast for a further 5–10 minutes until cooked through and golden brown.

Mix the chipotle paste with the mayo. Enjoy the popcorn cauliflower while hot with the mayo for dipping.

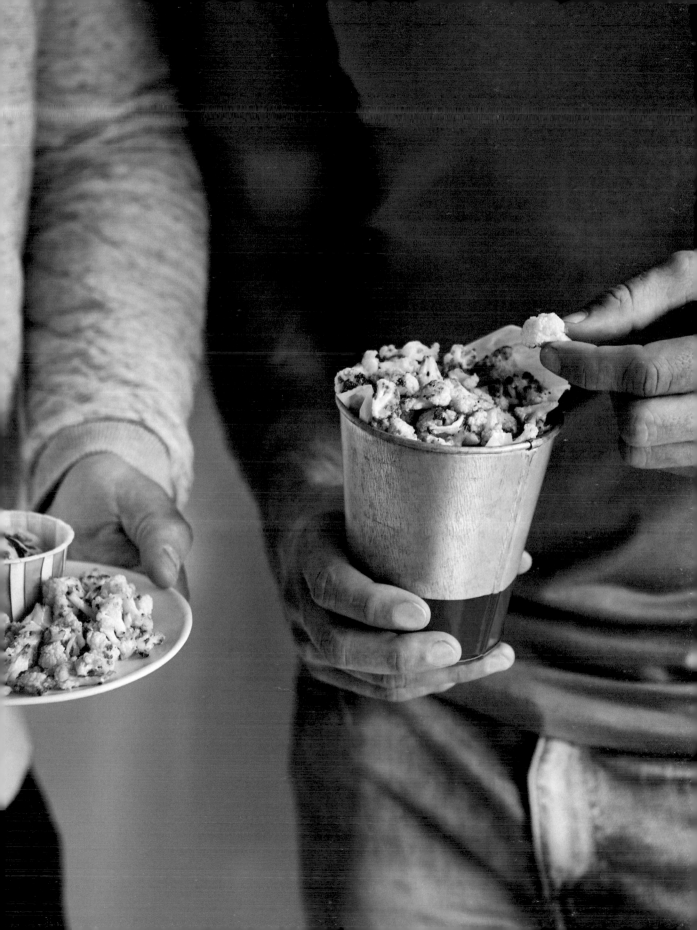

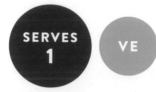

SERVES 1 **VE**

Beetroot and cumin hummus

MAKE AHEAD
Keep in an airtight container in the fridge for up to 3 days.

Ingredients

2 pre-cooked beetroots,
  drained and roughly chopped
150g chickpeas, drained
  and rinsed
½ tbsp tahini
½ tbsp olive oil
½ tsp ground cumin
squeeze of lemon juice
salt and pepper
carrot and cucumber sticks,
  to serve

Method

Put the beetroot, chickpeas, tahini, olive oil, cumin and a squeeze of lemon juice in a food processor and blitz until smooth. Season the hummus with salt and pepper to taste, adding more lemon juice if you like.

Serve with carrot and cucumber sticks.

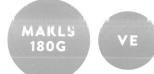

MAKES 180G **VE**

Curried roast chickpeas and coconut trail mix

**LONGER RECIPE
MAKE AHEAD**
Keep in an airtight container
for 1–2 days.

Ingredients

½ tbsp coconut oil

1 x 400g tin of chickpeas,
  drained and rinsed

1 tsp cumin seeds

salt and pepper

2 tbsp coconut flakes

1 tbsp mixed seeds

½–1 tbsp curry powder

1 tbsp sultanas

Method

Preheat the oven to 200°C (fan 180°C, gas mark 6).
Dollop the coconut oil into a high-sided roasting tray,
then transfer to the oven to heat up.

Transfer the rinsed chickpeas to a clean tea towel and
rub dry. Get rid of the skins that come off the chickpeas
as you rub them.

Carefully bring the hot roasting tray out of the oven. Tip
in the chickpeas and cumin seeds along with some salt and
pepper. Using oven gloves, shake the roasting tray to mix
everything together. Roast for 20–25 minutes until crisp.

While the chickpeas are roasting, toast the coconut flakes
and the mixed seeds in a dry frying pan over a medium heat
until the seeds pop. Take off the heat.

Come back to the cooked chickpeas. Take the tray out of
the oven and add the curry powder, toasted coconut flakes,
seeds and sultanas while still hot. Shake everything together,
then leave to cool.

Tomato, burrata and basil bruschetta

Ingredients

6 cherry tomatoes, halved –
  I like a mix of yellow and red
splash of red wine vinegar
drizzle of olive oil
salt and pepper
2 thick slices of baguette
1 clove garlic, peeled
50g burrata or buffalo
  mozzarella – make sure
  it is a veggie variety
a few basil leaves

Method

Mix the tomatoes in a bowl with the red wine vinegar, olive oil and a good pinch of salt and pepper. Leave to marinate for 5 minutes.

Toast the baguette, then rub each slice with the peeled garlic clove. Put onto a plate.

Top each slice of toast with the tomatoes, spooning over their juices, then tear the burrata or buffalo mozzarella and place on top. Scatter over a few basil leaves and enjoy.

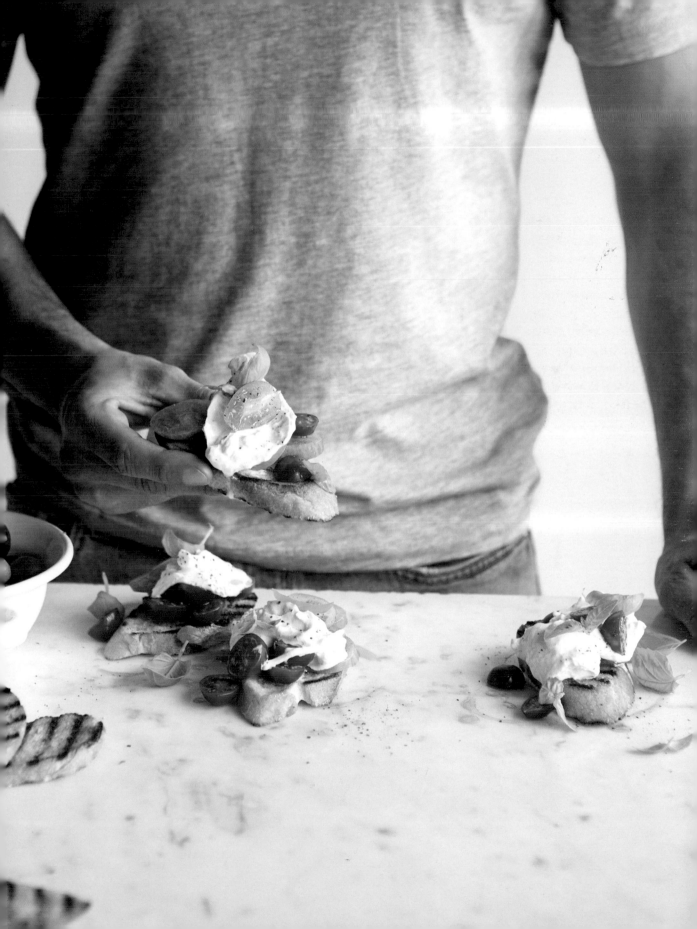

MAKES 4

Blueberry, poppy seed and lemon drop scones

Ingredients

70g self-raising flour
zest of 1 lemon
1 tsp poppy seeds
salt
50ml almond milk
1 egg
1 tbsp cooled melted butter,
   plus a smidge
2 handfuls of blueberries
honey, to serve

Method

Mix the flour, lemon zest and poppy seeds together in a bowl along with a small pinch of salt.

Pour the almond milk into a jug, then crack in the egg and add the melted butter. Whisk together.

Pour the wet ingredients into the dry. Give everything a good whisk until you have a smooth lump-free batter. Stir in the blueberries.

Melt a smidge of butter in a non-stick frying pan over a medium heat. Swirl it round to coat the base, then ladle in four drop scones with the batter. Fry the drop scones for about 90 seconds on each side. You will know when it is time to flip because they will be holding their shape and come away from the pan easily.

Serve warm. I like to spread mine with honey.

**MAKES
16**

**LONGER RECIPE
MAKE AHEAD**
Keep in an airtight container
for up to 1 week.

Ingredients

75g coconut oil, plus a smidge
100g medjool dates, pitted
  and roughly chopped
100g mixed seeds
1 ripe banana, peeled and
  roughly chopped
½ tsp bicarbonate of soda
200g rolled oats
1 scoop (30g) vanilla protein
  powder
salt

Seeded protein flapjacks

Method

Preheat the oven to 180°C (fan 160°C, gas mark 4).
Use a little coconut oil to grease a 20cm square loose-
bottomed brownie or cake tin, then line the base with
baking parchment.

Pour 100ml boiling water over the dates and give a little
stir to separate the fruit. Leave to soften for 5 minutes.

Meanwhile, toast the mixed seeds in a dry frying pan over
a medium heat, shaking the pan until they pop, then take
off the heat. Melt the coconut oil in the microwave.

Tip the soaked dates along with their water into a small
food processor with the melted coconut oil, banana and
bicarbonate of soda. Blitz until smooth, then scrape into
a bowl and mix in the oats, protein powder, toasted seeds
and a pinch of salt.

Tip into the lined tin, then use the back of a wooden
spoon to press into an even layer. Bake for 20 minutes
until golden and firm. Leave to cool in the tin, then cut
into sixteen squares.

SERVES 2

Coconut rice pudding with mango

LONGER RECIPE

Ingredients

75g pudding rice
1 x 400ml tin of coconut milk
2 tsp maple syrup
zest and juice of ½ lime
crushed seeds from
  2 cardamom pods
salt
1 scoop (30g) vanilla protein
  powder – optional
100g mango chunks

Method

Place the pudding rice, coconut milk, maple syrup, lime zest, crushed cardamom seeds, 100ml water and a pinch of salt into a saucepan. Give everything a good stir to combine, but don't worry if there are lumps of coconut as they will disintegrate while cooking.

Bring to the boil and simmer for 20–25 minutes, stirring regularly, especially towards the end when it will become creamy and thick.

Remove from the heat and leave to cool a little before stirring through the protein powder, if using.

Divide between two bowls, top with the mango chunks and lime juice. Eat the pudding straight away.

JOE'S TOP TIP Do not add the protein powder to the pan on the heat, or the whey will cook and go lumpy.

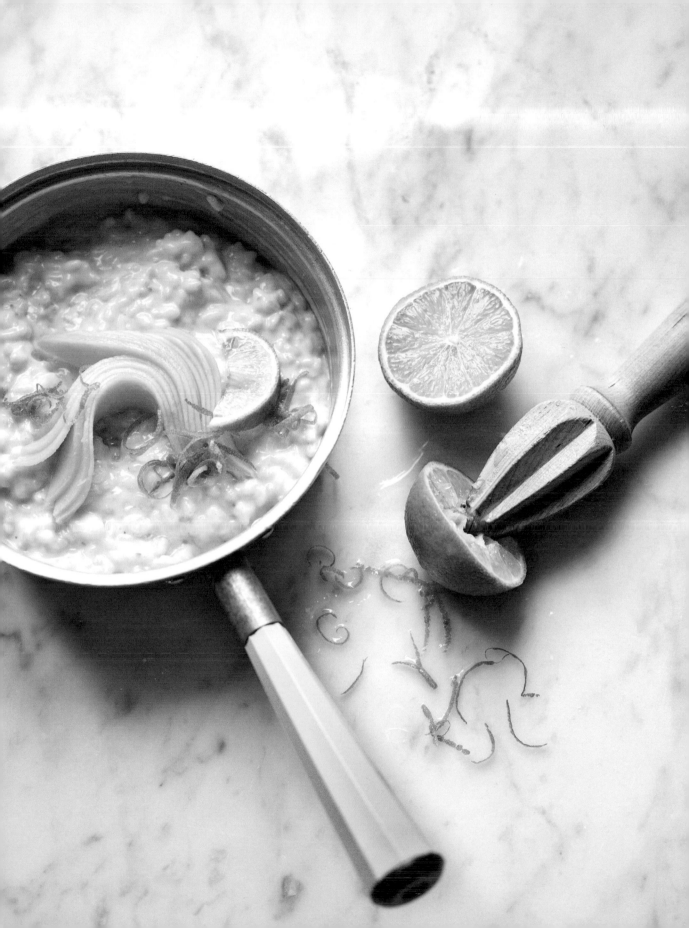

**LONGER RECIPE
MAKE AHEAD**
Cake only. Keep in an airtight
container for up to 3 days.
GOOD TO FREEZE
Cake only. When cooled, cover
well and keep in the freezer for
up to 1 month.

Ingredients

80g coconut oil, melted, plus
   a smidge for the tin
50g self-raising flour
100g ground almonds
2 scoops (60g) vanilla
   protein powder
1 tsp baking powder
1 tsp bicarbonate of soda
salt
80g cocoa powder (over 70%
   cocoa solids), plus more for
   dusting
150ml maple syrup
200ml coconut milk
zest of 1 orange
coconut yoghurt and
strawberries and/or raspberries,
   to serve – optional

Fantastic fudgy chocolate cake

Method

Preheat the oven to 160°C (fan 140°C, gas mark 3). Grease
a 20cm round cake tin with a little coconut oil and line the
base with baking parchment.

Mix the self-raising flour, ground almonds, vanilla protein
powder, baking powder, bicarbonate of soda and a pinch
of salt in a large bowl.

In a separate bowl, whisk the cocoa powder with 150ml boiling
water until well combined, then whisk in the melted coconut
oil, maple syrup, coconut milk and orange zest.

Pour the wet ingredients into the dry and give everything
a good whisk until you have a smooth runny batter. Pour into
the cake tin and bake for 35 minutes or until a skewer inserted
into the centre of the cake comes out clean.

Cool in the tin. When cool, dust with a little cocoa powder
and serve topped with coconut yoghurt and berries if
you like.

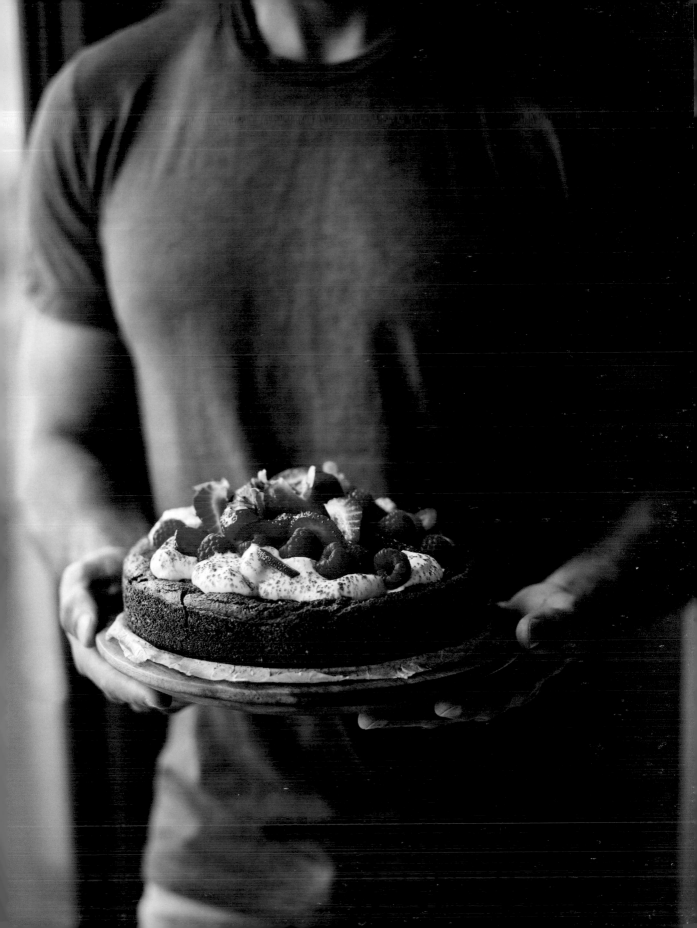

MAKE AHEAD
Keep in an airtight container
for up to 3 days.

GOOD TO FREEZE
Freeze before baking, then bake
from frozen, adding an extra
2 minutes to the cooking time.

Ingredients

100g peanut butter
1 tsp vanilla extract
3 tbsp maple syrup
1 egg
4 tbsp rolled oats
sea salt
50g raspberry jam

PBJ cookies

Method

Preheat the oven to 180°C (fan 160°C, gas mark 4) and
line two flat baking sheets with baking parchment.

Put all the ingredients apart from the jam in a bowl
and beat with a wooden spoon until you form a
smooth dough.

Dollop out mounded tablespoons of the mixture
(think Ferrero Rocher size) onto the baking sheets,
leaving space between each cookie as they will
spread in the oven.

Using your thumb, press into the middle of each cookie
to create a small well, then fill with a teaspoon of the jam.

Bake the cookies for 10–12 minutes until golden round
the edges. Cool on the tray for 5 minutes, then transfer
to a wire rack to cool completely. (Pictured overleaf.)

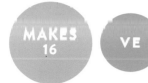

LONGER RECIPE
MAKE AHEAD
Keep in an airtight container
in the fridge for up to 1 week.

Ingredients

75g blanched hazelnuts
150g rich tea biscuits
75g coconut oil
200g dark chocolate (over
  70% cocoa solids)
2½ tbsp golden syrup
125g sultanas

Vegan rocky road

Method

Line a 20cm square loose-bottomed brownie or cake tin
with baking parchment.

Toast the hazelnuts in a dry frying pan until lightly golden
and smelling nutty, then allow to cool and roughly chop.

Put the rich tea biscuits in a ziplock bag (or if you don't have
one, leave them in the packet). Use the handle of a wooden
spoon to crush the biscuits into smaller rough pieces.

Break the chocolate into a large microwaveable bowl, then
spoon in the coconut oil and golden syrup. Zap in the
microwave in 30-second bursts, stirring in between, until
the chocolate has all melted.

Drop the crushed biscuits, chopped hazelnuts and
sultanas into the bowl and stir so everything is coated
in the chocolate mixture.

Tip the mixture into your tin, then use the back of a
wooden spoon to press the mixture down into an evenish
layer. Chill for 1–2 hours, until set.

When set, turn out and use a sharp knife to cut into sixteen
squares. (Pictured overleaf.)

**JOE'S
TOP TIP**   The mixture for these is so quick and easy
to make – just make sure to allow 1–2 hours
for setting in the fridge.

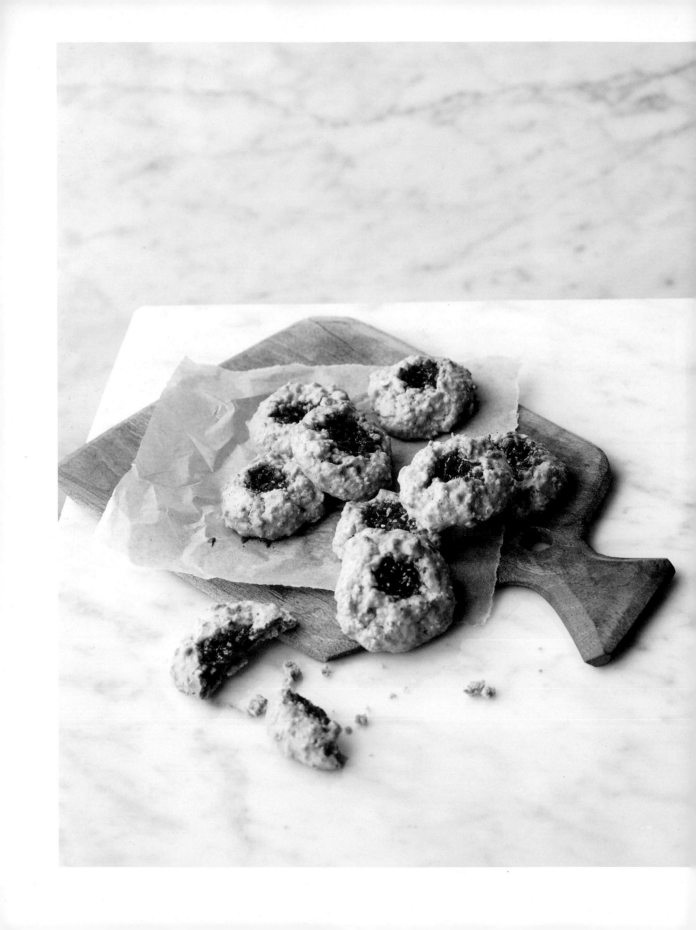

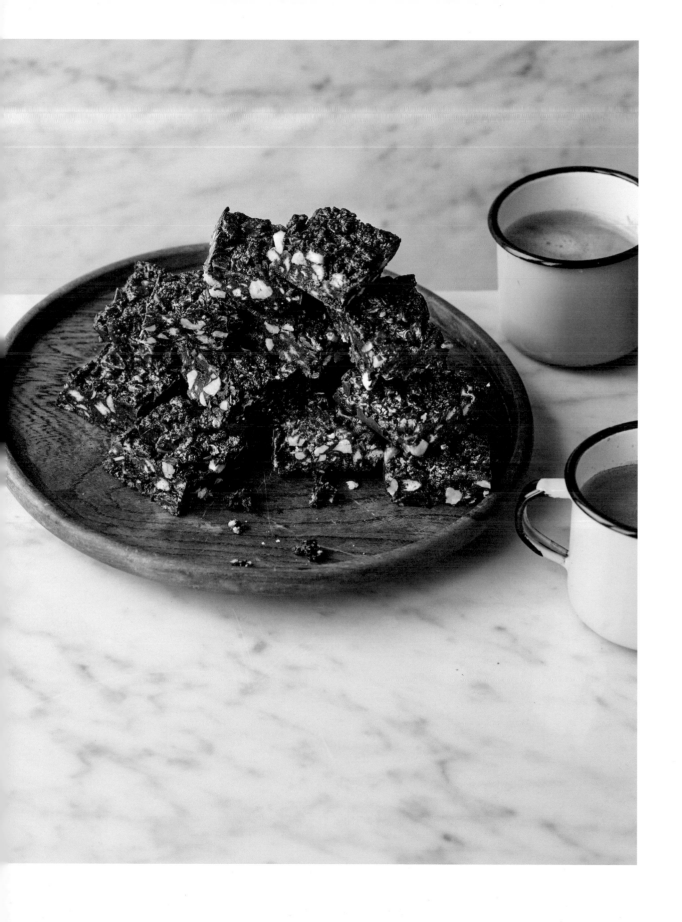

**MAKE AHEAD
GOOD TO FREEZE**
Freeze in the tray for up to 1 month.

Ingredients

**100g dark chocolate (over
70% cocoa solids)**
1 tsp coconut oil
½ tbsp maple syrup
**60g smooth peanut butter
(you want a natural
variety)**

Peanut butter cups

Method

Break the dark chocolate into a microwaveable bowl, add the coconut oil, then zap on high in 30-second bursts until the chocolate is melted.

Spoon 1 heaped teaspoon of the chocolate mixture into twelve holes of a round silicone ice cube tray – it needs to be silicone so that the peanut butter cups pop out easily.

Swirl the ice cube tray and use your teaspoon to coat the sides of each hole so that you are left with an even layer of chocolate covering the sides and base of each ice cube mould. This is the fiddly bit because you will have to go around the inside of each hole with your teaspoon a couple of times.

Place the ice cube tray in the freezer for 5 minutes to firm up.

Stir the maple syrup into your peanut butter. Take the ice cube tray out of the freezer, then spoon a teaspoon of the peanut butter into each hole. Smooth the top so it is flat, then spoon the remaining chocolate over each peanut butter cup to encase the filling. Put the tray back into the freezer.

When you want to eat one, simply pop it out of the ice cube tray, putting the rest back in the freezer. Leave for a couple of minutes to warm up slightly, then enjoy.

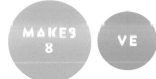

Salted 'caramel' chocolate truffles

LONGER RECIPE
MAKE AHEAD
Keep in an airtight container in the fridge for up to 1 week.
GOOD TO FREEZE
See tip below.

Ingredients

100g medjool dates, pitted and roughly chopped

2 tbsp cashew butter

½ tsp vanilla extract

2 tbsp coconut oil

1 tbsp cocoa powder (over 70% cocoa solids), plus 1 tbsp for rolling

sea salt

Method

Place the dates, cashew butter, vanilla extract, coconut oil, cocoa powder and a good pinch of salt in a small food processor.

Blitz until it comes together into a smooth paste. Roll into eight balls and place in the fridge for 1 hour, uncovered, to set.

Put the remaining 1 tablespoon of cocoa powder on a plate, then roll the truffles in it.

These freeze really well! Freeze on a tray in a single layer. This will stop them from clumping together. When frozen, transfer to a smaller more convenient container. Allow to defrost for 20–25 minutes before eating.

Caramelized banana split

Ingredients

10 pecan halves
1 small banana
1 tbsp butter
1 tbsp maple syrup
30g dark chocolate, broken
  into pieces
sea salt
1 spoonful of frozen yoghurt
  or your choice of ice cream

Method

Toast the pecans in a dry frying pan over a medium heat, then allow to cool and roughly chop. Cut your banana in half lengthways.

Put the frying pan back on the heat. Melt the butter, then stir in the maple syrup. Lay the banana cut-side down in the butter and syrup mixture. Cook for 3–4 minutes, regularly spooning the buttery syrup mixture over the banana to help it caramelize.

Ping the chocolate in the microwave for 30 seconds to melt it, then stir in a pinch of salt.

Put your caramelized banana slices, cut-side up, into a bowl. Spoon the frozen yoghurt or ice cream into the centre, then drizzle over the melted chocolate and sprinkle over the chopped pecans.

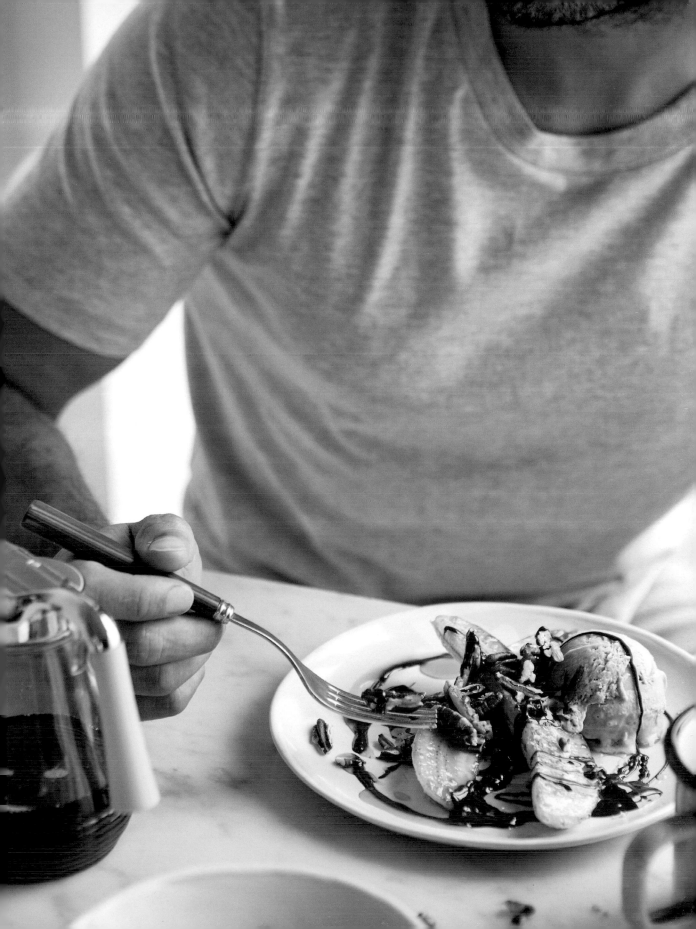

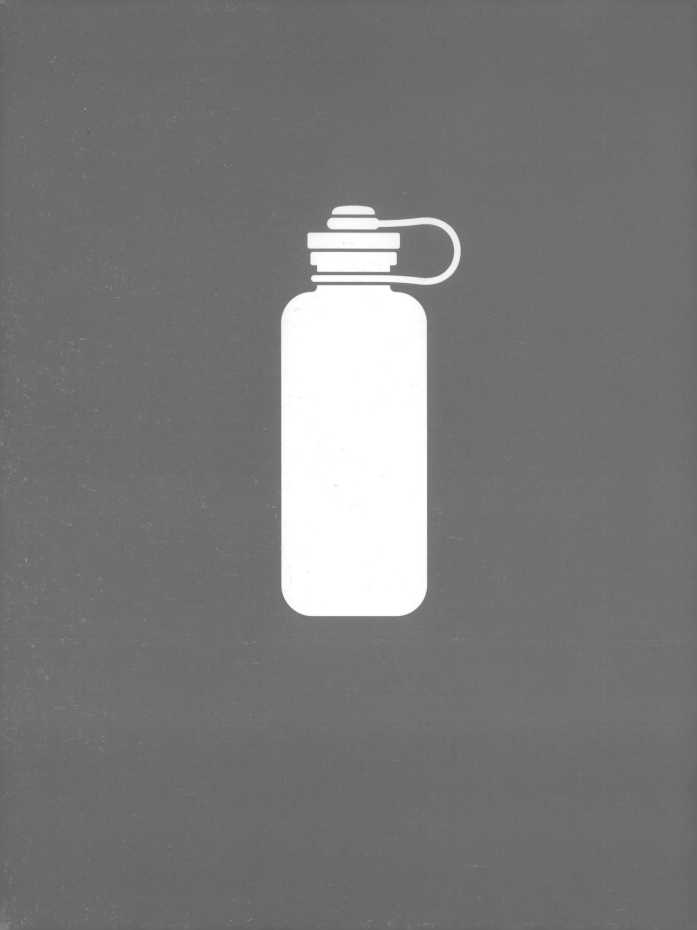

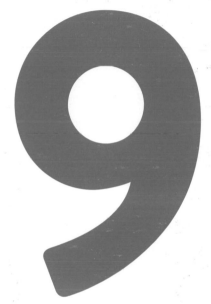

9

TRAINING

I am very passionate about about two things: food and fitness. I believe to have a healthy mind and body, you need to have a healthy attitude to both.

Luckily, my philosophy on food is almost the same as my philosophy with exercise: it should be quick, accessible and fun.

The biggest barrier people have to staying fit and healthy is time. But what if I said that you could get lean and fit with just 20–25 minutes of exercise a day? Would you be keen to give it a go?

This book contains recipes that take 15 minutes from start to finish. I am also including four workouts which can be done at home in under 25 minutes. If you want to try some of my free video workouts check out my YouTube Channel: The Body Coach TV.

I am a big proponent of short, intense home workouts. I believe training at home will increase your chance of success because with minimal equipment, space and time you can always squeeze in a daily workout and allow yourself to make progress. I've helped hundreds of thousands of people transform with nothing but a pair of dumbbells and their own bodyweight, so I believe I can do the same for you.

For this reason, I have designed four home workouts for you to combine alongside the recipes in this book. Three are full-body sessions targeting all the major muscle groups for a really great fat-burning effect and one focuses solely on strengthening your abs and core.

I suggest completing all four workouts in a week for a full, varied and challenging training routine. But if for example you love the kettlebell one, you could always do that twice a week and miss another one out.

Just a little reminder … Taking the easy option and only doing the abs workout four days a week is a sure-fire way to make very little fat-loss progress. The reality is, to build a strong, fit and lean body you need to work hard, so challenge yourself.

If you don't want to do any of the workouts in this plan and prefer to do spin classes, BodyPump, Boxercise, CrossFit or any other class, that's fine. Just be consistent and combine regular exercise with the healthy food in this book and sensible portion sizes, and you can't go wrong.

Be more active, every day

As well as the energy expended during a workout, there is also something called NEAT (Non Exercise Activity Thermogenesis). This refers to the amount of energy you expend throughout the day. For example: walking to work, taking the stairs, carrying your shopping bags to the car.

The more active you are in general, the more energy you will expend and the more body fat you will eventually burn.

Bodyweight HIIT

This workout is equipment-free, so you can utilize your own bodyweight to elevate your heart rate, improve your cardio and start to burn body fat.

Bodyweight workout

24 minutes
4 rounds
40 seconds work
20 seconds rest

1. Running sprints

Run up and down on the spot as fast as you can. Lift knees high, keep your back straight and pump your arms to accelerate.

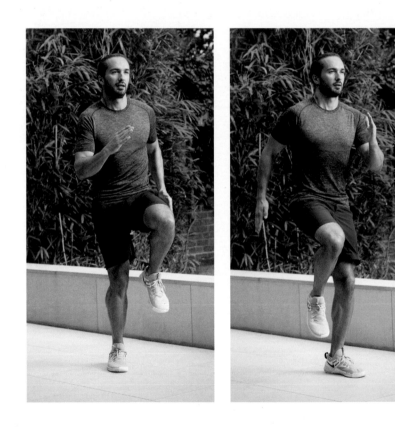

2. Mountain climbers

Start in a high plank position. Look down towards your hands and keep your back flat. Then drive your knees towards your chest as fast as possible.

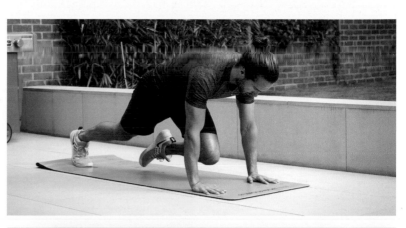

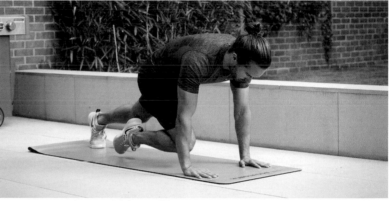

3. Squats

Place your feet in a comfortable position that will allow you to squat down while keeping them firmly flat on the ground. Sit low and drive through the heels to stand up. Repeat fast.

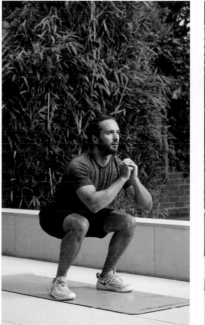

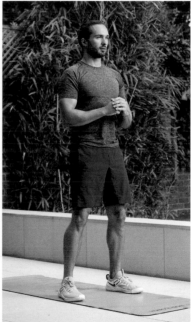

4. Lunges

Start with both feet together, then step forward with one foot and bend both knees into a lunge. Aim to keep your back straight. Alternate each leg.

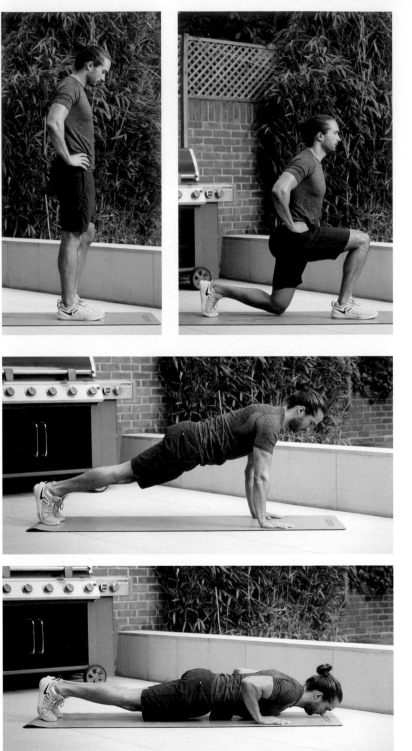

5. Press-ups

Start in a high plank position. Keep hands narrow and elbows close to the body. Lower yourself down towards the ground and push back up, fully extending your arms.

Alternative Spiderman

If you find standard press-ups too easy, then try this spiderman alternative. As you lower towards the ground, drive your knee out sideways towards your elbow. Beware: These are tough!

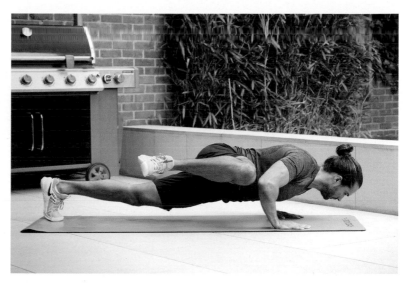

6. Burpees

Start standing, then place your hands on the floor in front of you. Quickly kick back your legs into a high plank, then lower your chest to the ground. Push up, jump feet forward and jump up into a standing position. Repeat as fast as you can.

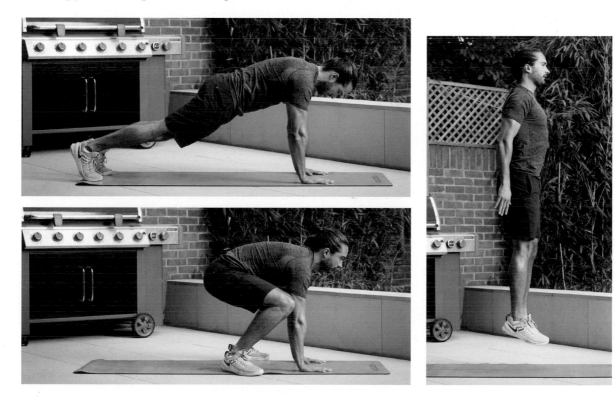

Kettlebell HIIT

A kettlebell is an awesome and inexpensive piece of kit. It's well worth the investment if you like to train at home. Most gyms also have a selection of kettlebells, so you could also follow this at the gym if you prefer. This workout is the most challenging one, aimed at improving your all-round physical conditioning. Your lungs will be working hard and your muscles will be burning, but the results are incredible.

Kettlebell workout

24 minutes
4 rounds
30 seconds work
30 seconds rest

1. Kettlebell swings

Stand with your feet shoulder-width apart and with the kettlebell in both hands. Keep your back straight and swing the kettlebell to eye level. Do this by slightly bending the knees but mainly hinging from the hips to thrust forward and create momentum.

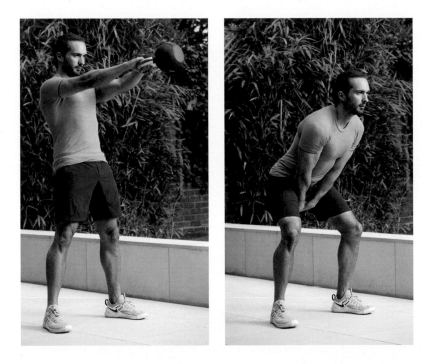

2. Goblet squats

Hold the kettlebell in both hands close to the chest as you lower down into a squat. Aim to keep your core engaged and back straight.

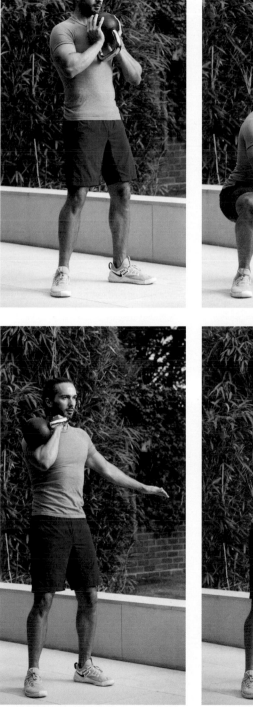

3. Single-arm military press

Rack the kettlebell up high onto your arm. Then drive the kettle bell upwards until your arm is fully extended. Use the same arm for one round, then swap arms on the next round.

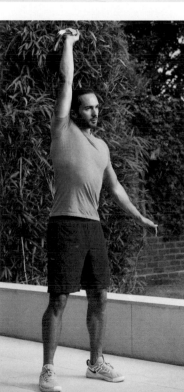

4. Reverse lunges

Rack the kettlebell up high on one arm. Start with feet together, then step one foot backwards into a reverse lunge. Repeat the lunges on the same leg for one round, then change legs and swap arms on the next round.

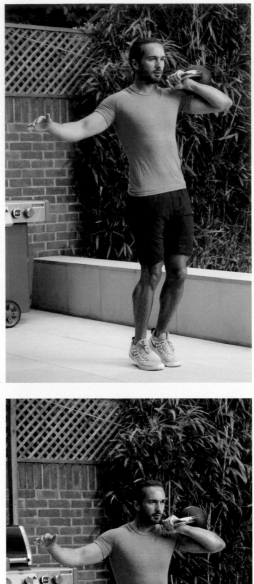

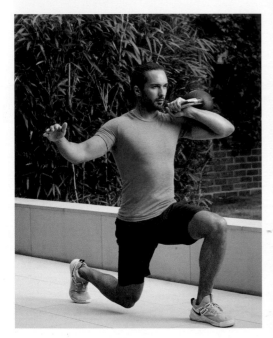

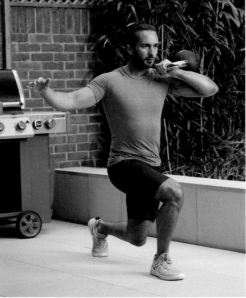

5. Dead lifts

Hold the kettlebell in both hands, keep a slight bend in knees and hinge from the hips to lower the kettlebell towards the ground. Focus on using your hamstrings and glutes to pull the kettle back up to a standing position.

6. Single-arm thrusters

Hold the kettlebell in one hand and rack it up high on your arm. Lower down into a squat and as you come up, drive the kettlebell into a shoulder press. Rest it back on the arm, squat and repeat. Alternate the arm on each round.

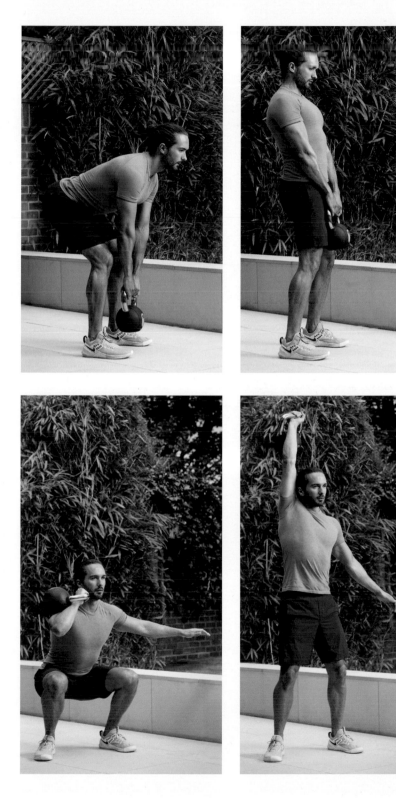

Dumbbell HIIT

This can help build lean muscle through resistance training. This will focus on upper-body and lower-body exercises by adding weights into the mix. The important thing to note here is to choose weights that are challenging and each week aim to progress with heavier ones. This will result in muscle hypertrophy (when new muscle is built). In turn this will increase your metabolism and get your body burning more energy.

Dumbbell workout

24 minutes
4 rounds
30 seconds work
30 seconds rest

1. Bicep curls

Standing up straight with one dumbbell in each hand, one at a time slowly curl up each dumbbell towards your shoulder. Rotate the hand as you curl each dumbbell.

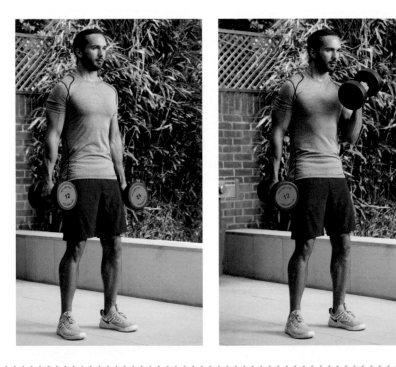

2. Front squats with weights

Rack the dumbells up high on the front of your shoulders. Keep your core engaged as you lower down into a squat. Drive through the heels back up into a standing position and repeat.

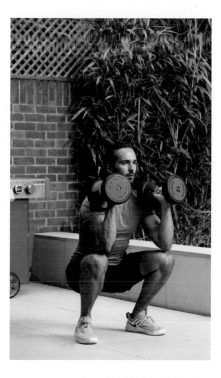

3. Dead lifts

Hold one dumbbell in each hand. Keep a slight bend in your knees and hinge from the hips to lower the dumbbells towards the ground. Focus on using your hamstrings and glutes to return to a standing position.

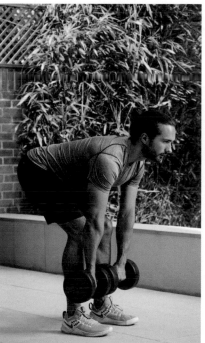
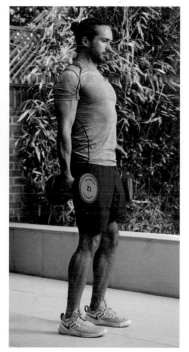

4. Shoulder press

Hold one dumbbell in each hand with elbows pointing out. Then drive the hands up until the dumbbells meet. Slowly lower and repeat in a controlled way.

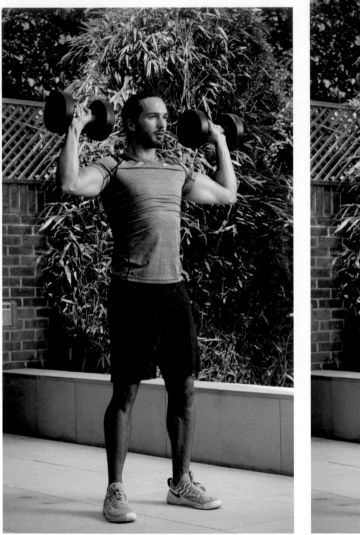
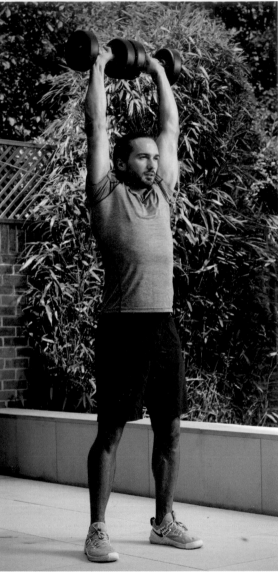

5. Weighted step-ups

Find a box step, bench or low wall to step onto. Hold one dumbbell in each hand. Step one foot up onto the step and drive the other knee up towards your chest. Step down and repeat with alternating legs.

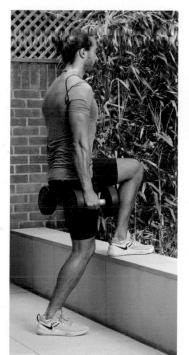

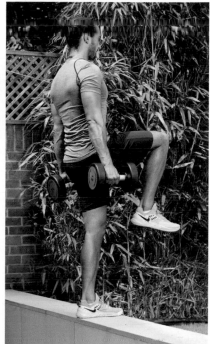

6. Tricep dips with weight

Place a weight securely between your thighs. Keeping elbows tucked in, lower yourself towards the ground, then push back up to fully extend your arms.

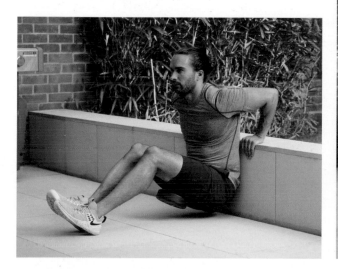

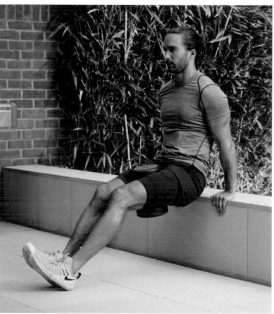

Abs circuit

Everyone loves an abs and core workout. However, don't be under the illusion that only doing an abs workout and avoiding the others will suddenly result in a six-pack. This workout is less strenuous and will not burn many calories at all. The only way you will get visible abs is if you reduce your body-fat levels. That's achieved by creating an energy deficit through the more intense cardio and resistance training workouts.

Abs circuit

24 minutes
4 rounds
40 seconds work
20 seconds rest

1. Crunches

Lie down with your knees bent with both feet flat on the floor. Move your hands to your temples and slowly crunch up towards your knees. Repeat for 40 seconds.

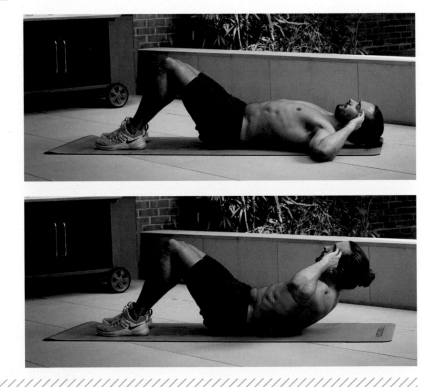

2. Toe touches

Elevate your legs straight up in the air. Crunch up and try to touch your toes or shins.

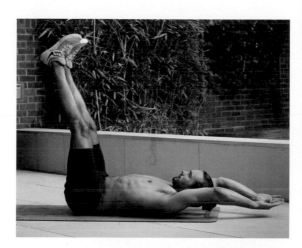

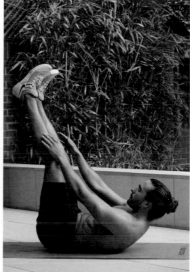

3. Bicycle crunches

Place your hands on your temples. As you crunch, try to twist so your opposite elbow touches your opposite knee.

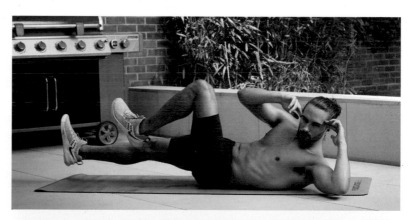

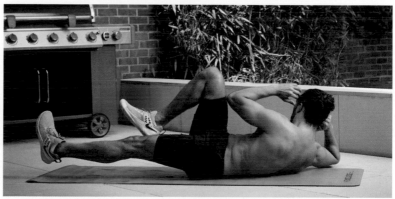

4. Leg raises

Raise your shoulders slightly off the ground to engage your abs. Lower your legs straight ahead until your heels are about 15cm from the ground. Using your abs, pull your legs back up and repeat.

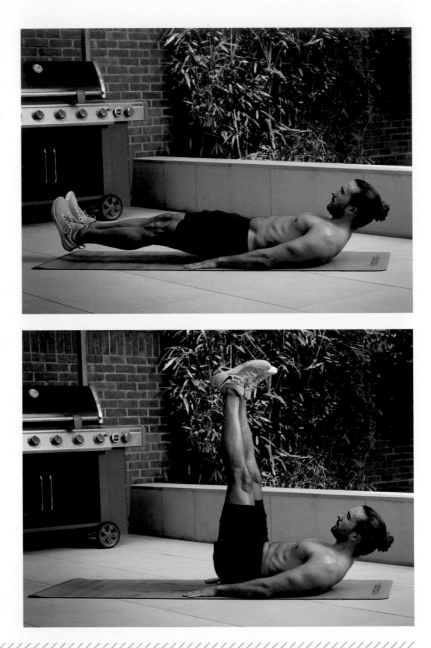

5. Plank

Lift and hold your torso and legs off the ground with your elbows on the floor directly under your shoulders. Aim to keep a flat back and active abs and glutes.

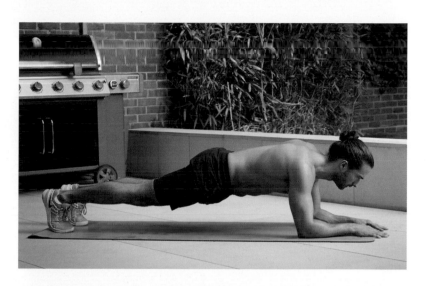

6. Side plank

Place one elbow on the ground directly under your shoulder. Keep a straight line from your feet to your shoulder. Lift up and hold. Alternate sides each round.

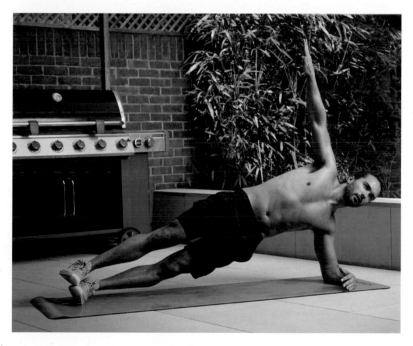

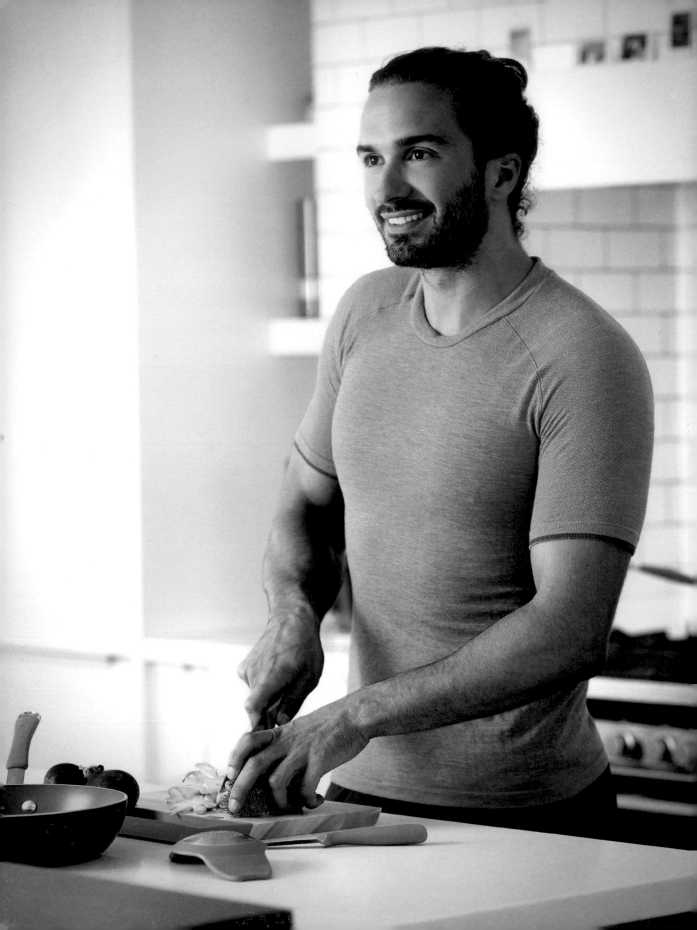

Acknowledgements

I would like to start by saying a big thank you for your support, whether you follow me on social media, complete my YouTube workouts or invest in my cookbooks. I love sharing content and I feel really proud to have built such a strong community online, with the shared goal of everyone getting fitter, healthier and happier.

I'd like to thank everyone at Bluebird for giving me the chance to produce another wonderful book which I'm so proud of. I think *Veggie Lean in 15* will improve the lives of many around the world and have a big impact on people's health and fitness.

Thanks as always to my photography and styling team, Maja and Bianca, who always work so hard and help turn my simple recipes into beautiful images that people want to cook.

And one big thank you to all my friends and family who always support and encourage me to achieve more and keep my feet firmly on the ground.

Lots of Love, Joe

Index

Note: page numbers in *italics* refer to illustrations.
Recipes in **bold** refer to vegan dishes.

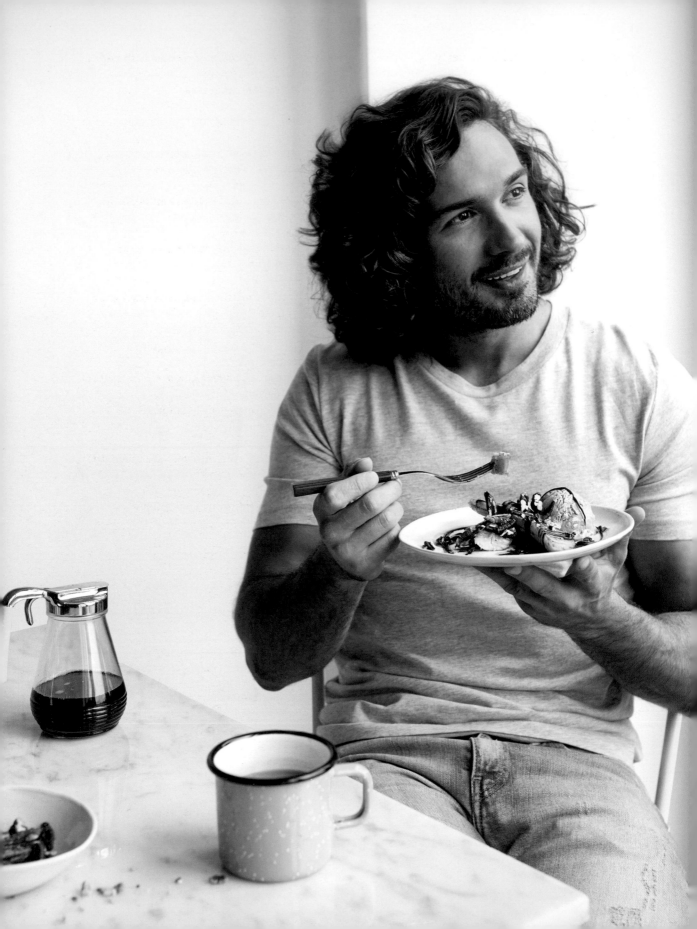

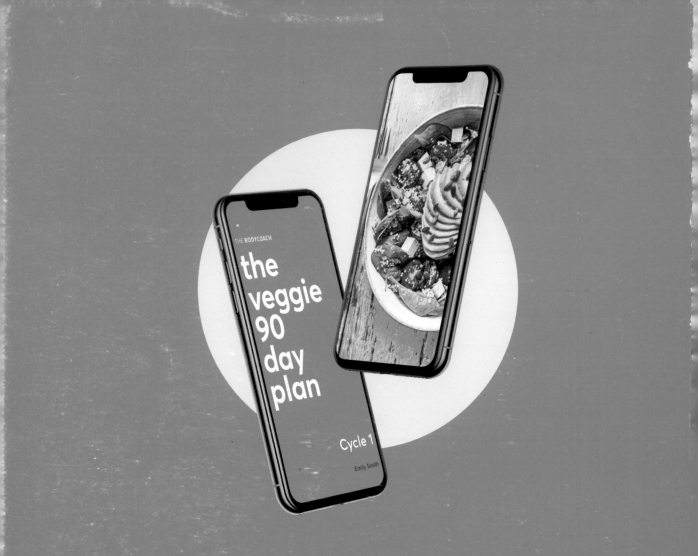

The All New Veggie 90 Day Plan

With new and tasty vegetarian recipes, the all new Veggie 90 Day Plan is now available. This tailored plan will give you all the tools you need - including 15 real-time workouts and access to our exclusive Facebook support group - to transform your body and become fitter, stronger, healthier and leaner than you've ever been.

Get started at **www.thebodycoach.com**